Generalized Anxiety Disorder:
Diagnosis, Treatment and its Relationship to Other Anxiety Disorders

3rd Edition

Generalized Anxiety Disorder:
Diagnosis, Treatment and its Relationship to Other Anxiety Disorders

3rd Edition

David Nutt, DM, MRCP, FRCPsych
Professor of Psychopharmacology

Spilios Argyropoulos, MSc, MRCPsych
Clinical Lecturer in Psychiatry

Sam Forshall, MRCPsych
Consultant Psychiatrist

Psychopharmacology Unit
School of Medical Sciences
University of Bristol
Bristol, UK

MARTIN DUNITZ

First published in the United Kingdom in 1998 by Martin Dunitz Ltd,
The Livery House, 7–9 Pratt Street, London NW1 0AE

Tel.: +44 (0) 20 7482 2202
Fax.: +44 (0) 20 7267 0159
E-mail: info.dunitz@tandf.co.uk
Website: http://www.dunitz.co.uk

Third edition 2001

Although every effort has been made to ensure that drug doses and other information are presented accurately in this publication, the ultimate responsibility rests with the prescribing physician. Neither the publishers nor the authors can be held responsible for errors or for any consequences arising from the use of information contained herein. For detailed prescribing information or instructions on the use of any product or procedure discussed herein, please consult the prescribing information or instructional material issued by the manufacturer.

Distributed in the USA by:
Fulfilment Center, Taylor & Francis, 7625 Empire Drive,
Florence, KY 41042, USA
Toll Free Tel: 1-800-634-7064 Email: cserve@routledge_ny.com

Distributed in Canada by:
Taylor & Francis, 74 Rolark Drive, Scarborough, Ontario M1R 4G2, Canada
Toll Free Tel: 1-877-226-2237 Email: tal_fran@istar.ca

Distributed in the rest of the world by:
ITPS Limited, Cheriton House, North Way, Andover,
Hampshire SP10 5BE, UK
Tel: +44 (0) 1264 332424 Email: reception@itps.co.uk

A CIP record for this book is available from the British Library.

ISBN 1-84184-135-8

Printed and bound in Italy by Printer Trento S.r.l.

Contents

The concept of generalized anxiety disorder. Historical introduction

The mental and physical symptoms that are currently included under the anxiety disorders have been observed for centuries (Table 1). During the first half of the 1800s, the individual physical symptoms were considered to be specific diseases of the heart, inner ear, gastrointestinal system and other systems of the body. Each symptom was taken at face value and the physicians attempted to treat them as real physical complaints. Meanwhile, the mental component of anxiety was usually seen as part of the melancholic state.[1] Darwin though, in 'The Origin of Species', differentiated anxiety from depression. He linked the former with the anticipation of future experiences and the latter with past ones.

Table 1
Evolution of the concept of anxiety disorders

1800s	Independent symptoms
1866	Morel — one syndrome
1894	Freud
1964	Klein — different syndromes
1980	DSM-III
1992	ICD-10
1994	DSM-IV

As the century progressed, the idea that these symptoms may be the diverse manifestations of a unitary syndrome/ concept called anxiety gradually evolved. Feuchtersleben in 1847[1] was the first to view anxiety as a cause of organic disease, of the heart and digestive system in particular, hence re-establishing the link between mind and body. Morel, in 1866, making use of the newly formed concept of the autonomic nervous system, proposed that changes in this system may give rise to mental symptoms ('emotional delusions'). He thus tried to explain a clustering of symptoms hitherto seen as unrelated.

In 1894, Freud finally brought these diverse symptoms together in his seminal paper 'The justification for detaching from neurasthenia a particular syndrome: the anxiety neurosis'.[2] At that time the traditional neuroses, i.e. hysteria and hypochondriasis, were considered psychological in origin, while obsessional states and the new 'anxiety neurosis' were thought, even by Freud, to have an organic basis. This unitary view remained dominant throughout most of the 20th century, despite disagreements on the nature of anxiety, which led to different therapeutic approaches. Some attempts to remove panic and social phobia from the fold went largely unnoticed.

It must be emphasized that the development of the above ideas was largely based on clinical observations and psychopathological insights, without hard scientific evidence. In 1964, Klein[3] was the first to produce such evidence. Based on differential responses to pharmacological treatment, in that panic attacks were reduced with imipramine but free floating anxiety was not, he argued for the extrapolation of panic disorder from the general syndrome of anxiety. Similar arguments for social phobia followed a few years later. Despite counter-arguments, these views were gradually incorporated into the modern classification systems, beginning with DSM-III in 1980.

The subsequent surge of interest and research into panic disorder and, to a lesser extent, social phobia left generalized anxiety disorder (GAD) as an essentially residual diagnosis ascribed to patients who did not fulfil the criteria for any of the other, more specific, anxiety disorders. In recent years, the interest in this 'forgotten' category has resurfaced, largely owing to new insights into the epidemiology and neurobiology of anxiety as well as the advent of new effective treatments.

The evolution of the concept of generalized anxiety from the sociological point of view is also interesting. Clark[4] argues that, with the coming of industrialization over the last 200 years, many of the traditional causes of acute anxiety and panic in society, e.g. famines and large epidemics, began to recede allowing more insidious causes of individual anxiety to become prominent. The change in the basic conditions of existence meant that anxiety and panic were no longer seen as continuous features of everyday life but as avoidable disturbances of mental health and general wellbeing. It is therefore under this light that they acquired specific clinical significance.

Diagnosis, classification and epidemiology of GAD

Classification

With the publication of the third edition of the Diagnostic and Statistical Manual of Mental Disorders (DSM-III)[5] in 1980 the concept of anxiety neurosis was abandoned, and GAD was differentiated from panic disorder. The diagnosis of GAD in DSM-III required the presence of persistent generalized anxiety for at least 1 month. In addition to this, its diagnosis required symptoms from at least three of four categories that included motor tension, autonomic hyperactivity, apprehensive expectation and vigilance and scanning. However, it was essentially a residual diagnosis, for, owing to the hierarchical structure of DSM-III, GAD could not be diagnosed if patients met criteria for another disorder.

The publication of DSM-III-R[6] brought substantial changes and, in particular, the hierarchical exclusion rules were modified so that GAD could be diagnosed, except where there was a coexisting mood or psychotic disorder. Psychic anxiety was defined in terms of excessive or unrealistic worry in two or more areas and not related to another Axis I disorder. The somatic symptoms criteria were changed to the presence of at least 6 of 18 somatic symptoms that formed three clusters:

motor tension, autonomic hyperactivity, and vigilance and scanning. Importantly, the duration period was extended from 1 to 6 months, so further differentiating it from an adjustment disorder. With these changes, GAD became an independent diagnosis.

As a result of field trial data, DSM-IV[7] introduced further revisions (Table 2). The core feature is of excessive anxiety about a number of events occurring on more days than not for a period of at least 6 months. In addition, the anxiety must be perceived as being uncontrollable, and must not be confined to features of another Axis I disorder (e.g. anxiety relating to panic attacks in panic disorder). There was further revision of the somatic symptoms, with 3 of the 6 symptoms of restlessness, fatiguability, impaired concentration, irritability, muscle tension and sleep disturbance being required. For the diagnosis to be made, the disorder must cause clinically significant distress or impaired functioning. In DSM-IV, as in DSM-III-R, GAD cannot be diagnosed where it occurs exclusively in conjunction with a mood or psychotic disorder.

The ICD 10 classification[8] also includes the diagnosis of GAD, and like DSM-IV uses the criteria of a 6 month duration, but in other respects differs significantly (Table 3). Unlike DSM-IV, the worry does not have to be excessive or seem uncontrollable. Furthermore, there is a significantly greater emphasis on autonomic hyperarousal, and the requirement of at least 4 of 22 somatic symptoms. In ICD-10 GAD there are no criteria relating to distress or impairment.

In summary, for the clinical diagnosis of GAD, the core feature is the presence of excessive worry. This is felt to be uncontrollable and it must cause significant impairment. The anxiety should not relate to another Axis I disorder and must be accompanied by 3 of 6 somatic symptoms.

Table 2
DSM-IV criteria for generalized anxiety disorder.

A. Excessive anxiety and worry (apprehensive expectation), occurring more days than not for at least 6 months, about a number of events of activities (such as work or school performance).

B. The person finds it difficult to control the worry.

C. The anxiety and worry are associated with three (or more) of the following six symptoms (with at least some symptoms present for more days than not for the past 6 months). Note: Only one item is required in children.

(1) restlessness or feeling keyed up or on edge

(2) being easily fatigued

(3) difficulty concentrating or mind going blank

(4) irritability

(5) muscle tension

(6) sleep disturbance (difficulty falling or staying asleep, or restless unsatisfying sleep)

D. The focus of the anxiety and worry is not confined to features of an Axis I disorder, e.g., the anxiety or worry is not about having a Panic Attack (as in Panic Disorder), being embarrassed in public (as in Social Phobia), being contaminated (as in Obsessive-Compulsive Disorder), being away from home or close relatives (as in Separation Anxiety), gaining weight (as in Anorexia Nervosa), having multiple physical complaints (as in Somatization Disorder), or having a serious illness (as in Hypochondriasis), and the anxiety and worry do not occur exclusively during Post Traumatic Stress Disorder.

E. The anxiety, worry, or physical symptoms cause clinically significant distress or impairment in social, occupational or other important areas of functioning.

F. The disturbance is not due to the direct physiological effects of a substance (e.g., a drug of abuse, a medication) or a general medical condition (e.g., hyperthyroidism) and does not occur exclusively during a Mood Disorder, a Psychotic Disorder, or a Pervasive Developmental Disorder.

Table 3
ICD-10 criteria for generalized anxiety disorder.

A. There must have been a period of at least 6 months with prominent tension, worry, and feelings of apprehension about everyday events and problems.

B. At least four of the symptoms listed below much be present, at least one of which must be from items (1) to (4):

Autonomic Arousal Symptoms

(1) palpitations or pounding heart, or accelerated heart rate;
(2) sweating;
(3) trembling or shaking;
(4) dry mouth (not due to medication or dehydration);

Symptoms involving chest and abdomen

(5) difficulty in breathing;
(6) feeling of choking;
(7) chest pain or discomfort;
(8) nausea or abdominal distress (e.g., churning in stomach);

Symptoms involving mental state

(9) feeling dizzy, unsteady, faint or lightheaded;
(10) feelings that objects are unreal (derealization), or that the self is distant or 'not really here' (depersonalization);
(11) fear of losing control, 'going crazy', or passing out;
(12) fear of dying;

General symptoms

(13) hot flushes or cold chills
(14) numbness or tingling sensations;

Symptoms of tension

(15) muscle tension or aches and pains;
(16) restlessness and inability to relax;
(17) feeling keyed up, on edge, or mentally tense;
(18) a sensation of lump in the throat, or difficulty in swallowing;

Cont'd.

ICD-10 criteria–continued

Other non-specific symptoms

(19) exaggerated response to minor surprises or being startled;

(20) difficulty in concentrating, or mind 'going blank', because of worrying or anxiety;

(21) persistent irritability;

(22) difficulty in getting to sleep because of worrying;

C. The disorder does not meet the criteria for panic disorder, phobic anxiety disorders, OCD, or hypochondriacal disorder.

D. Most commonly used exclusion clause. The anxiety disorder is not due to a physical disorder, such as hyperthyroidism, an organic mental disorder, or a psychoactive substance-related disorder, such as an excess consumption of amphetamine-like substances or withdrawal from benzodiazepines.

Clinical presentation

GAD is characterized by both psychological and physical symptoms. The psychological symptoms that dominate its presentation are a persistent feeling of fearful anticipation, irritability, poor concentration, and a feeling of restlessness. Patients often complain of a poor memory, but this is secondary to impaired concentration. While the repetitive worrying thoughts tend to be of everyday matters, they can also be focused on physical symptoms. For example, where autonomic hyperarousal is present, a patient may be aware of his heart beat and worry about an incipient heart attack.

The physical symptoms stem from two principal sources, muscle tension and autonomic hyperarousal. Muscle tension may cause tremor and muscle aches particularly in the back and shoulders. In addition it can cause tension headaches, which are felt as a bilateral constriction or pressure, especially in the frontal or occipital regions. Autonomic hyperarousal can affect every body system causing numerous associated somatic symptoms. For example, respiratory symptoms may include a feeling of tightness in the chest and overbreathing, while cardiovascular symptoms include palpitations, and chest pains. Not infrequently it is the physical symptoms of anxiety that are the presenting complaint, especially in general practice.

Atypical presentations

In GAD, because somatic symptoms may be prominent, patients often seek medical rather than psychiatric help. In one study, twice as many sought a medical rather than a psychiatric opinion.[9] As a result, GAD patients frequently present in specialist medical clinics with unexplained physical symptoms. A high proportion of patients with non coronary chest pain have GAD. For example it was found that GAD patients equalled those with panic disorder in a cardiology clinic.[10] Some 40% had been investigated with an exercise ECG, while 33% had been investigated with an echocardiogram. Another study found that 23% of patients with atypical chest pain in an emergency department were suffering with GAD.[11] An investigation of 216 patients with chest pain but normal coronary angiograms found that over 50% had a diagnosis of GAD compared with 20% with panic disorder.[12] In a survey of 50 patients with DSM-III GAD, 48% had a history of chest pains and, of these, 87% reported that chest pain was not related to panic attacks.[13] Other common atypical presentations include irritable bowel syndrome, and hyperventilation syndrome. In a small study, 82% of GAD patients met criteria for the hyperventilation syndrome,[14] while another study found that 25% of GAD patients could induce their symptoms by voluntary hyperventilation.[15]

Differential diagnosis

The symptoms of GAD can arise in many different conditions and its diagnosis is further complicated by comorbidity. GAD must be distinguished from anxiety due to a medical disorder. Numerous medical conditions, for example hyperthyroidism, cause symptoms of anxiety (Table 4). These are diagnosed on the basis of the history, physical examination and laboratory investigations.

Table 4
Medical conditions causing symptoms of anxiety.

Cardiovascular conditions	Neurological conditions
Angina pectoris	Akathisia
Arrhythmia	Mass lesion
Valvular disease	Epilepsy
Endocrine conditions	**Respiratory disease**
Hypercalcaemia	Asthma
Hyperthyroidism	Chronic obstructive airway disease
Carcinoid	Pulmonary embolism
Metabolic conditions	
Hyperkalaemia	
Hypoglycaemia	
Hyponatraemia	
Hypoxia	
Porphyria	

Furthermore, GAD has to be distinguished from substance-induced anxiety. Numerous substances can cause anxiety, including toxins and drugs of abuse as well as prescribed medication (Table 5). In particular, there is considerable overlap between the symptoms of GAD and alcohol withdrawal. In both conditions anxiety, agitation, poor concentration and irritability are prominent features. However, their respective time courses differ. In GAD, these symptoms are enduring and not only related to a reduction or cessation of prolonged heavy drinking. Moreover, in alcohol withdrawal, autonomic hyperactivity is more prominent and the condition can be complicated by confusion, hallucinations and seizures.

Excessive anxiety is common to all other anxiety disorders and GAD must be differentiated from these (Table 6). In contrast to GAD, in other anxiety disorders worry is focused on a particular aspect of their psychopathology. For example, in social phobia the anxiety is focused on being embarrassed in public, while in hypochondriasis anxiety is focused on having a serious physical illness. Excessive worry is also a key fea-

Table 5
Medications causing symptoms of anxiety.

Amphetamines
Anticholinergics
Antihypertensives (e.g. reserpine, hydralazine)
Antituberculous drugs (e.g. isoniazid)
Caffeine
Digitalis (toxicity)
Sympathomimetics (e.g. ephedrine, pseudoephedrine)
Levodopa
Neuroleptics (akathisia)
Bronchodilators (e.g. salbutamol, theophylline)
Thyroid hormones
Non-steroidal anti-inflammatory agents
Selective Serotonin Re-uptake Inhibitors

Table 6
Generalized anxiety disorder symptom overlap.

	GAD	Panic	Depression
Anxiety and worry	X	X	X
Panic attacks		X	
Poor concentration	X	X	X
Irritability	X		X
Sleep disturbance	X	X	X
Depressed affect			X
Hyperarousal	X		X
Motor tension	X	X	X

ture of obsessive-compulsive disorder (OCD), but while in GAD the worry concerns everyday matters, in OCD it relates to egodystonic intrusive thoughts, which can also take the form of urges or impulses, and are often accompanied by compulsions. The performance of the compulsive act diminishes the anxiety, albeit temporarily.

Anxiety is a frequent accompaniment of depression, which can be differentiated by the presence of a depressed affect. GAD cannot be diagnosed where it only occurs in the course of a mood disorder or psychotic disorder.

Finally, GAD needs to be differentiated from 'normal worry'. Although both 'normal worry' and GAD involve a preoccupation with everyday concerns, certain features discriminate the two. In contrast to non-pathological anxiety, the worry in GAD is pervasive, distressing and enduring. It results in significant interference with functioning and is more likely to be accompanied by physical symptoms.

The epidemiology of GAD

Demography

Epidemiological research gives few consistent findings with respect to the demography of GAD (Table 7). The Epidemiological Catchment Area (ECA) study,[16] using DSM-III criteria, found that it was more common among women and young people (under the age of 30). It tended to be more prevalent in urban areas and amongst those with lower incomes, but there was no clear association with standard of education.

Another major USA epidemiological study, the National Comorbidity Survey (NCS),[17] which used DSM-III-R criteria, confirmed that it was more common in women, but in contrast to the ECA study found that it was more common in those aged over 24. Like the ECA study, GAD was correlated with lower income groups, although this did not reach significance following adjustment for covariants. The NCS also found that GAD correlated with those who had previously been married (as opposed to those who were married or had never been married), thus replicating the previous finding that GAD was more common in those divorced, widowed or separated.[18] Other correlates in the NCS included homemakers and the unemployed, which included a high number of those permanently disabled and early retirees.

Table 7
Demographic characteristics of generalized anxiety disorder sufferers.

Female (67%)
Previously married
Homemakers
Unemployed
Lower income
Urban dwellers
Neuroticism

Finally, there is a body of research that suggests that those with anxiety neurosis, which includes GAD, have a preponderance of neurotic personality traits. In a study that followed over 3000 male conscripts for 17 years, it was found that compared with controls, those with anxiety neurosis differed strongly on the following dimensions: nervousness, depressiveness, frustration tolerance, inhibition and neuroticism.[19] Other research has produced similar findings.[20,21]

Prevalence

The changing diagnostic criteria of GAD, particularly those regarding its duration and hierarchical position, mean that surveys of its prevalence vary in their findings. For example, in a survey of 357 women, the prevalence of GAD was 11.5% using the 1 month criterion, but only 2.4% if the 6-month criterion was employed.[22] Following the introduction of DSM-III, several community surveys found current prevalence in the range 1.2%–6.4%, while lifetime prevalence ranged from 4%–6.6%. A survey of over 3000 households found GAD to be the most common psychiatric disorder with a 1 year prevalence of 6.4%.[23] The first DSM-III based longitudinal epidemiological study, which followed a cohort of nearly 600 19 and 20 year olds, over a 7 year period, found that 1 year prevalence of GAD was stable across time, with rates fluctuating between 1.3% and 2.0%. Finally, the ECA study,[16] which only examined for GAD in three of its five centres, found GAD to be a common disorder with a reported lifetime prevalence of 4.1%–6.6%.

There have been two regional surveys reporting on the prevalence of GAD using DSM-III-R criteria. In Florence it was found that the prevalence of current GAD was 2%, and that of lifetime GAD was 3.9%.[24] In Basel the lifetime prevalence of GAD was found to be 1.9%, but the prevalence was four times greater than this when the ICD 10 criteria were applied.[25] The NCS,[17] which applied a structured interview to a representative US national sample, found the current, 12 month and lifetime rates of GAD to be 1.6%, 3.1% and 5.1% respectively. As in other studies, rates were higher where ICD 10 criteria were applied, with the lifetime prevalence being 8.9%. This reflects the difference between the DSM and ICD criteria, the former being more stringent.

High rates of GAD have also been found in both children and the elderly.[26] A 1 year prevalence rate of 2.9% was found for 'overanxious anxiety disorder' — the childhood equivalent of GAD. Even higher rates were found in adolescents. In the elderly, GAD has consistently been found to be the most prevalent of the anxiety disorders with rates varying between 0.7% and 7.1%.[27]

High prevalence rates have also been found in the primary care setting. When 330 patients were examined in four primary care centres, a prevalence rate of 10% was found, which compared with a rate of 11% for panic disorder.[28] Another study found that 6.4% or primary care patients met the full syndrome of GAD, while 12% of patients had symptoms but did not meet the full criteria.[29]

In summary, while there has been a considerable variation in the prevalence rates found, GAD is consistently one of the most common anxiety disorders, both in community and primary care surveys as well as in all age groups.

Comorbidity

Psychiatric comorbidity

Population surveys have found comorbid diagnosis to be very common in GAD (Table 8). Indeed in some studies over 90% of GAD patients met the criteria for at least one other

Table 8
Psychiatric comorbidity rates of GAD.

Diagnosis	Percentage
Simple phobias	21–55
Pure GAD	10–26
Social phobia	15–59
Depression (including dysthymia)	8–39
Panic disorder	3–27

concurrent disorder.[26] In children, overanxious disorder is found to have concurrent comorbidity rates of over 50%.[30] This finding lends support to the idea that overanxious disorder is a prodromal form of GAD.

The ECA study[16] found comorbidity rates of 58%–65%, with panic disorder and major depression being the most common comorbid diagnoses. A longitudinal epidemiological study of a cohort in Zurich found a strong association between GAD and depression, but a lower association of GAD with panic.[19] In addition, patients who suffered with comorbid conditions had greater functional impairment and, importantly, a high risk of attempted suicide. The NCS[17] found that 66.3% of those with current GAD had another comorbid diagnosis, whereas 90% of those with a lifetime diagnosis of GAD had at least one other psychiatric disorder. Like the ECA study, the most frequent comorbid disorders were mood and panic disorders.

Thus, 'pure' GAD is a relatively rare disorder. This has led some authorities to question the validity of GAD as an independent diagnosis, suggesting that it may be the prodrome, epiphenomenon, or residual of other disorders. However, in the NCS, a third of GAD sufferers carried no other concurrent or recent diagnosis. For those with comorbid illness, it was found that they were both more severely ill, and were more impaired. Furthermore, treatment was more complicated and had a worse outcome.

Comorbidity with alcohol problems

Generally, anxiety disorders are found to have high rates of comorbidity with alcohol problems. It was found, using the DSM-III diagnosis of anxiety neurosis, which includes both GAD and panic disorder, that up to 25% of sufferers have alcohol problems.[31] Of inpatients with alcohol problems, 8.3%–56.2% also had a history of GAD, the great variation reflecting differing diagnostic criteria. When those with GAD are surveyed for alcohol problems, 9%–15% have a history of abuse. In a review of the epidemiology of GAD it is concluded that alcoholism is less prevalent than in other anxiety disorders.[26] Furthermore, those with GAD described a pattern of abuse that was brief and non-persistent, and which tended to occur during the early adult years. In contrast to other anxiety disorders, it was found that in 60% of cases alcohol problems either preceded or were synchronous with the onset of GAD.[32] This is consistent with the finding that prolonged heavy drinking acts to increase levels of anxiety. Both acute and chronic pathological alcohol consumption may produce symptoms that mimic anxiety states and may sensitize individuals to their own somatic responses.[31] In addition, the negative social, legal and familial consequences of long-term alcohol abuse may substantially increase stress, anxiety and worry. However, anxiety symptoms also function to motivate drinking as a source of symptom relief. Therefore it would seem that, as with other anxiety disorders, the relationship between GAD and alcohol is a transactional one.

Medical comorbidity

GAD and medical illness interact with one another in three separate ways. Firstly, the physical illness can directly cause symptoms of anxiety, e.g. hyperthyroidism. Secondly, the symptoms of anxiety can be misdiagnosed as having been caused by medical illness, e.g. in atypical chest pain. Finally, medical illness can be a focus of worry and psychological anxiety.

It is likely that GAD is prevalent in many medical conditions, but there is relatively little research in this area.[33] Most of this research has not used structured diagnostic interviews and, moreover, is difficult to interpret because of the changes in diagnostic criteria. Thus, in a study of acute stroke patients 24% of subjects met the criteria for GAD,[34] while in patients 2–3 months post-stroke the prevalence was only 3%.[35] This would imply that the former study was in fact diagnosing an adjustment disorder, from which DSM-III GAD was poorly differentiated. Four diagnoses that have high levels of comorbidity with GAD are irritable bowel syndrome,[36] ulcerative colitis,[37] diabetes mellitus[38] and chronic fatigue syndrome.[39] Prevalence rates in patients with irritable bowel syndrome range from 20%–37%. Furthermore, it was found that, with the effective treatment of anxiety, the bowel symptoms improved as well. With respect to chronic fatigue syndrome, which is characterized by fatigue lasting more than 6 months, over 50% of sufferers met the criteria for GAD.

The validity of the diagnosis of GAD

There are a number of problems with GAD as a diagnostic entity. It has the lowest inter-rater reliability of all the anxiety disorders.[40] In addition, it has the highest rates of comorbidity both with respect to depression and other anxiety disorders.[26] This has led critics of the concept to argue that it is not an independent diagnosis but merely a prodrome, epiphenomenon or residual state of other disorders with which it coexists. Others regard it as a vulnerability factor for other anxiety or mood disorders. In a robust defence of the concept, it is argued that, far from being a mere epiphenomenon of other disorders, in many respects GAD can be considered the 'basic anxiety disorder' because its defining features, anxious expectation and hyperarousal, reflect the basic processes of anxiety.[40] Unlike the other anxiety disorders, it has no clear behavioural marker to facilitate its differentiation and it is this that reduces inter-rater reliability. Furthermore, it is argued that high comorbidity is a feature of all anxiety disorders, with rates of comorbid diagnosis averaging about 50%, and over 70% in the case of panic disorder. While it is acknowledged that comorbidity is common in GAD some 20%–26% may have 'pure' GAD.

It may be that there are aspects of the current diagnostic criteria (DSM-IV and ICD-10) that do lack validity. When demographic and comorbidity profiles of patients with varying levels of anxiety pathology were examined both in terms of duration and numbers of symptoms, it was found that time, whether 1 month or 6 months, was less discriminating than the symptom profile.[41] Thus subjects with six or more symptoms of anxiety produced a particular epidemiological profile. These subjects were characterized as being younger, single, with low household income, and relatively low educational attainment. Further evidence that the number of symptoms present may be important to the validity of the diagnosis is provided by an examination of the characteristics of familial (DSM-III-R) GAD in twins.[42] It was found that individuals with a high familial vulnerability for GAD, as reflected by the risk of GAD in their co-twin, systematically differed in their clinical characteristics compared with those with low vulnerability. The strongest predictor of risk of illness in the co-twin was the number of symptoms endorsed. Therefore, it may be that the validity of GAD would be increased if a larger number of symptoms were required to meet the diagnostic criteria. It may be the case that, in DSM-IV, by reducing the number of symptoms required to make the diagnosis, the validity of the diagnosis has been reduced.

Course, prognosis, disability and costs

The course of GAD

The onset of GAD tends to be both insidious and early.[19] The Epidemiological Catchment Area (ECA) study found the median age of inception to be the early 20s.[16] In addition it was found to be common in children and adolescents, in whom the mean age of onset was 10 years.[43] In a follow-up study of 164 patients with GAD, it was found that the mean age of onset was 21 years.[44] However, the NCS[17] found the onset to be common after the age of 25. Consistent with this, is the finding that the average age of presentation for treatment was approximately 39 years.

While the evidence concerning the onset of the illness is in some respects conflicting, evidence concerning its course is consistent (Table 9) and mostly points to it being chronic and

Table 9
The course of GAD.

Insidious onset
Onset in 20s
Course: chronic and recurrent
Remission rate is low

recurrent.[45] The ECA study[16] found that half of those with a life-time history of GAD were ill at the time of interview. In 40% of cases the illness was found to have a duration of over 5 years, with a mean duration of 6–10 years. In another study[44] the average duration of illness was greater than 20 years, and on average patients rated themselves to be symptomatic for 56% of their lives. Consistent with high levels of chronicity is the finding of low rates of remission. In the same study, in which the subjects were followed up over a period of 3 years, remission rates were identified. At 1 year the rate was 15%, while at 2 years it had risen to only 25%. Remission rates were substantially lower where GAD was comorbid with another anxiety disorder. Most patients were found to remain with a stable level of symptoms, but relapse rates were high in those whose symptoms had remitted. Of those who achieved a full symptomatic remission, 15% had relapsed within 1 year. The risk of relapse was greater both where the remission was partial and for those whose GAD had been comorbid with another disorder. In this case, annual relapse rates were about 25%. Furthermore, outcome appears still worse when psychiatric inpatients are examined. In this population, recovery rates of 15%–18% were found during follow-up over 4–8 years.[19] In a longitudinal cohort study,[19] where patients were followed up for up to 9 years, recovery rates were about 25%, with about 60% of patients remaining subjectively impaired at work or in other social roles. Again, in this study, those with comorbid disorders had a worse outcome.

Prognosis

Given that GAD tends to have a chronic course with low rates of recovery, the conclusion must be drawn that the prognosis is, by and large, unfavourable. Longitudinal studies suggest that most patients still suffer from symptoms, and over half are functionally impaired after many years.

There are few predictors of outcome in GAD (Table 10). There is however a general rule for all studies predicting the outcome of mental disorders: 'that course is best predicted by former course' (Angst). This seems to be the case in GAD. There are other factors that suggest a poor outcome. Firstly, comorbidity is associated with lower remission rates. Secondly, there is evidence that when GAD is coexistent with a longstanding somatic disorder the outcome tends to be worse. There is a body of evidence suggesting that coexistent personality disorder predicts a worse long-term outcome for neurotic disorders generally.[46] In addition personality disorder has an unfavourable influence on treatment outcome.[47] Finally, the quality of social adjustment, and marital and family relationships in neurotic disorder, have been found to be at least as important as clinical factors in predicting outcome.[48]

Table 10
Predictors of poor prognosis in GAD.

Long duration of illness
Comorbid psychiatric disorder
Longstanding somatic disorder
Coexistent personality disorder
Poor social adjustment
Poor marital and family relationships

Disability and GAD

There is a widespread belief that GAD, in contrast to other disorders, is not associated with significant disability or dysfunction. In short, sufferers are dismissed as being the 'worried well', with the implication that they really should not be troubling their doctor. In fact, research presents a very different picture. The NCS[17] found that 28% of those with GAD alone, and 51% of those with comorbid GAD, had symptoms that interfered with their life activities. A study that compared patients with GAD and those with panic disorder using the Clarke Personal and Social Adjustment Scale[49] found that it was the former who were more disabled. Another study, using the Sheehan Disability Scale, found that patients with GAD were at the threshold between mild and moderate impairment, and thus were comparable to those with uncomplicated panic disorder.[50]

These findings are endorsed by a study which assessed the quality of life of 357 subjects with DSM-III-R GAD and/or panic disorder.[51] It was found that 9% of subjects had made a suicide attempt, with no significant difference between diagnostic groups. Patients with GAD rated their emotional health worse than those with panic disorder alone. In terms of functional activity, those with GAD were significantly disabled, with 25% receiving disability benefit and over a third receiving public assistance. Only slightly more than 50% were in fulltime employment. A substantial number (43%) reported impaired social functioning, and functional impairment was generally greater where conditions were comorbid.

Thus GAD causes significant interference in its sufferers' lives. This is borne out by the finding reported in the NCS[17] that 66% of subjects had sought professional help, and 44% had used medication to treat the illness.

The cost of GAD

It can be seen that GAD comes at a considerable cost to the individual as a result of significant functional impairment, but what of the wider cost to society as a whole?

There has been no research into the economic cost of GAD specifically, although there has been research into the cost of the anxiety disorders as a whole. The human capital approach has been used to estimate both the direct costs (reflecting the cost of treating the disorder) and the indirect costs (consisting of the lost productivity caused by the disorder).[52] Anxiety disorders are common, and it is estimated that they consume over 30% of mental health costs in the USA. If costs are proportionately attributed to diagnosis according to prevalence, then it would be predicted that GAD consumes nearly 6% of the mental health budget. In fact, this is probably an overestimate for two reasons. Firstly, the cost of treating each case is probably significantly lower for GAD than certain other disorders, e.g. obsessive-compulsive disorder. Secondly, research in the primary care setting indicates that, because GAD has an early onset and a chronic course, it tends to be under diagnosed.[53] Moreover, where a diagnosis is made, treatment is often not offered. Thus the direct cost of treatment is probably lower than would be expected given the high levels of morbidity found in community surveys. However, it is estimated that only 23% of the total cost of the disorder is represented by treatment costs, and over 75% of the cost to the economy takes the form of lost productivity (Figure 1).[52] This is clearly illustrated in a study which demonstrated that over a third of GAD sufferers were maintained on benefits, and only a little over half the subjects were in fulltime employment.[51] Some 38% reported that they had lost more than a week of work in the past year as a result of their difficulties.

In addition to both the direct and indirect costs, there are other hidden costs relating to GAD. As has already been discussed, patients are frequently seen in general medical clinics where they present with unexplained physical symptoms. Often they have been extensively and expensively investigated before being referred to psychiatrists. For exam-

Figure 1
Costs of GAD: the iceberg.

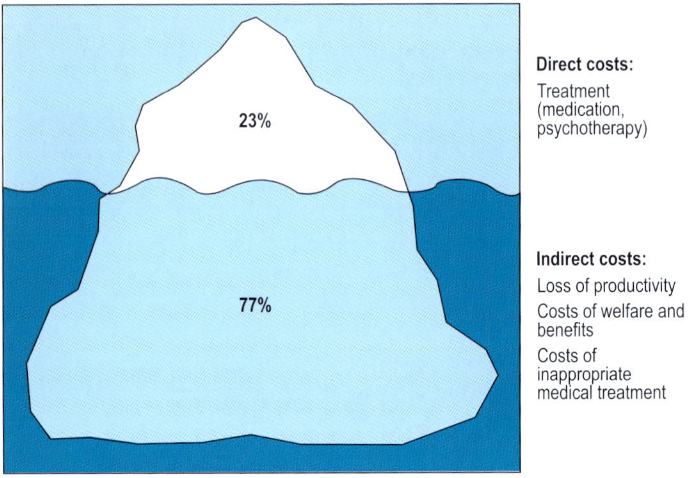

ple it was found that 71 patients with anxiety neurosis referred to psychiatrists, who had first been investigated by general physicians, had been subjected to 358 tests and procedures (5 per patient), and 135 speciality referrals (almost 2 per patient).[54] Thus in addition to the direct cost of treatment there is often costly and inappropriate utilisation of health resources. This is confirmed in a study that looked at 119 high health care users in a large health maintenance organization in Seattle.[55] Of these, 40% had a life history of GAD, 22% had GAD as a current diagnosis, of which 9% had 'pure' GAD.

Thus the bulk of the cost relating to GAD does not involve its treatment, but relates to the impairment that is secondary to the condition. It is tempting to hypothesize that, with more accurate diagnosis and effective treatment, the overall cost of the illness would fall sharply.

Causation and mechanisms of GAD

Genetic studies

A twin study[56] found no evidence for genetic transmission of GAD. A high frequency of non-anxiety psychiatric disorders in co-twins was observed. This indicates that GAD is probably aetiologically heterogenous. A second twin study[57] was also negative, showing that genes contributed to the predisposition of personality traits, but not to specific diagnoses of GAD or panic. However, a third twin study[58] produced a concordance for GAD among monozygotic twins versus dizygotic twins of 4.3:1, thus suggesting a genetic influence. Further, another study[59] reported an increased rate of GAD (but not other anxiety disorders) in the first degree relatives of patients. Therefore, there may be a degree of familial transmission of the condition and differentiation from other anxiety disorders, such as panic,[60] while GAD and depression appear to share, to a degree, the same genes.[61]

Genetic causation, at least in part, is further supported by the recent finding that a polymorphism in the serotonin transporter gene, which results in functional abnormality of the reuptake of this transmitter from the synaptic cleft back to the cell (Figure 2), accounts for a small percentage of anxiety related personality traits in individuals and their siblings.[62]

Figure 2
Serotonergic neuron and receptors. 5HT-1A (pre- and postsynaptic) and 5HT-2 are implicated in GAD.

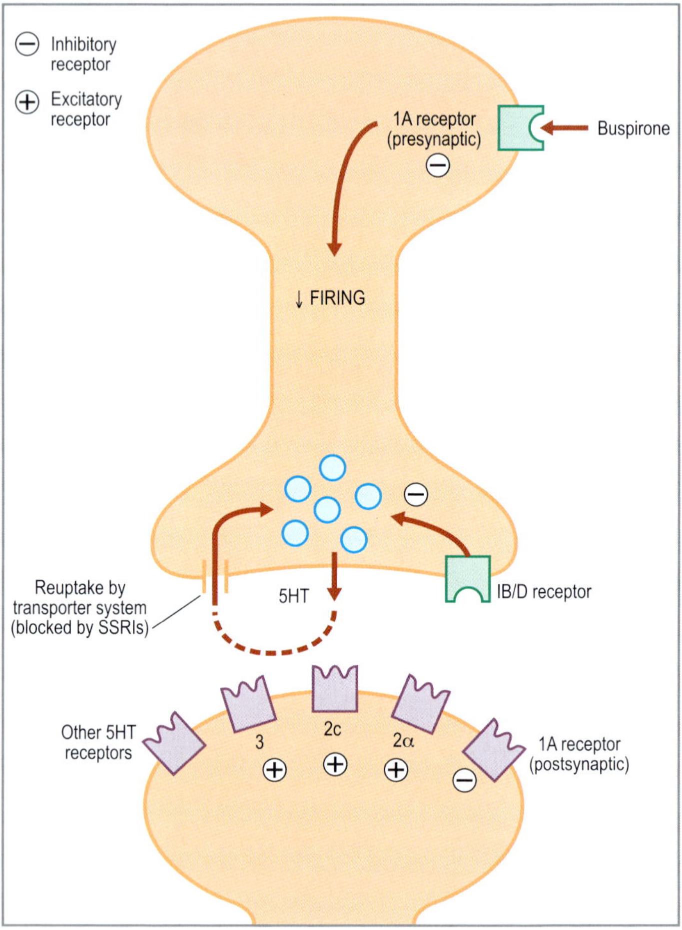

Neurobiology

A variety of methods can be applied in the study of the neurobiology of psychiatric disorders, and a number of them have already been tested in GAD (Table 11). The brain as a whole, or specific regions that are thought to be implicated in a particular condition, are investigated using neuroimaging techniques, both at rest and during activation paradigms that attempt to mimic or provoke the condition in question. Changes in the glucose metabolic rate, the regional or global blood flow, and oxygen utilization are useful indicators of anatomical and functional abnormalities.

At the neurochemical level, neurotransmitter systems can also be tested for evidence of baseline abnormality or for dysfunction during challenge tests that specifically activate the system in question. A similar approach is used for the neuroendrocrine system. Finally, manifestations of baseline or activation abnormalities are sought in a variety of peripheral neurophysiological parameters. An overview of the methods applied in GAD and the results obtained so far appear in Table 11.

Functional neuroanatomy

There are very few imaging studies so far in patients with GAD, but they suggest potential changes in global and regional activity in this population.

At rest, the global or regional blood flow does not differ significantly between GAD patients and normal controls. However, in state anxiety, a decrease is observed in cerebral blood flow in most brain regions.[63]

The baseline metabolic rate can be measured by cerebral glucose metabolism using positron emission tomography (PET). In one such study with GAD patients, their metabolic rate was higher, compared with normal controls, in parts of the occipital, temporal and frontal lobes, the cerebellum and thalamus. Meanwhile there was a decrease in other areas of the temporal lobe, the basal ganglia and the cingulate gyrus.

Table 11
Ways of studying the neurobiology and psychiatric disorders applied in GAD.

	Test	GAD
Neuroanatomy	R. blood flow	At rest: normal In stress: ↓
	Metabolic rate	At rest: ↑ ↓ In stress: ↑ (basal ganglia)
Neurochemistry		
GABA	Saccadic eye movements	↓ receptor sensitivity
	Platelets & lymphocytes	↓ receptor sensitivity
	SPET	↓ receptor binding (left temporal pole)
5HT	CSF levels	↓
	Challenge (m-CPP)	↑ anxiety/anger
NA	Plasma levels	Normal
	MHPG	Normal
	MAO-A/COMT	Normal
	Challenge (clonidine)	Blunted GH response
CCK	Challenge (pentagastrin)	Induces panic
Neuroendocrinology		
HPA axis	Cortisol levels	Normal
	Challenge (DST)	38% abnormal
Neurophysiology	Autonomic responses	At rest: normal, but ↑ muscle tension In stress: weaker responses, slower recovery Abnormality: ? ↓ autonomic flexibility,

Cont'd.

Neurophysiology (continued)		
		? ↓ parasympathetic activity
	EEG	At rest: equivocal
		In tasks: ↑ vigilance
	Psychophysiological	↓ fine motor activity
		↓ reaction time
		↓ critical flicker frequency
	Sleep	↓ total sleep
		↓ sleep efficiency
		↓ slow wave sleep
		Initial/middle insomnia

During a vigilance task there was a relative increase in the metabolic rate in the basal ganglia and the right parietal lobe, but not in the limbic area or the cortex. Finally, treatment with benzodiazepines resulted in a decrease in the metabolism in the occipital cortex, limbic system and basal ganglia.[64,65]

Overall, the picture is still somewhat confusing, but the above findings point towards an involvement of several cortical regions plus the basal ganglia in generalized anxiety. The above data suggest that, similar to obsessive-compulsive disorder, there may be hyperactive brain circuits in GAD (Figure 3), whereas in depression the circuits are underactive. Further, the increase in metabolic activity observed in the thalamus may account for hypervigilance, a prominent symptom in GAD.[66]

Neurochemistry

Gamma-aminobutyric acid (GABA)

This is the main inhibitory neurotransmitter in the brain. When GABA receptors are blocked anxiety rises, and

Figure 3
A neuroanatomical model of GAD. Brain circuits, symptoms and neurotransmitter sites of drug action.

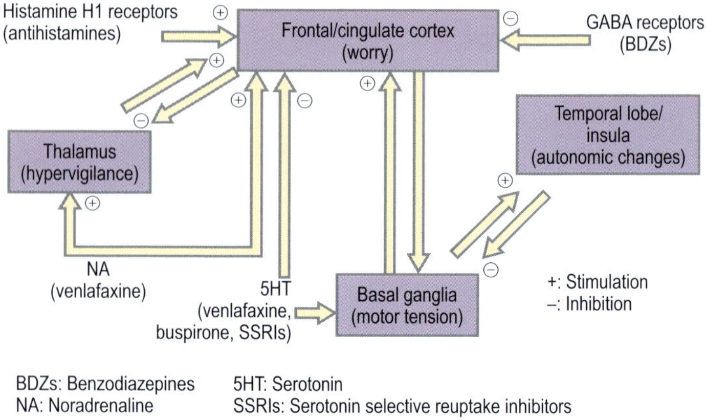

when they are stimulated, e.g. by benzodiazepines, it falls (Figure 4). The sensitivity of central benzodiazepine receptors is studied by measuring the velocity of the saccadic eye movements. In GAD, reduced sensitivity of these receptors has been reported,[67] although less conclusively compared with panic disorder.

Decreased sensitivity of platelet and lymphocyte benzodiazepine receptors is also found in GAD. After treatment with diazepam the receptor binding returns to normal.[68,69]

Tiihonen et al[70] used single photon emission tomography (SPET) with a new benzodiazepine receptor radioligand, [123]NNC 13-8241, to compare the receptor binding between 10 patients with GAD and an equal number of healthy volunteers. They reported a significant decrease in the left temporal pole, a finding also reported in patients with panic disorder.[71] Unlike panic, however, there was no increase in binding in the right prefrontal cortex. The authors suggest that their finding further differentiates GAD from panic, and

Figure 4
The role of the GABA-A receptor in anxiety. Actions which mimic or potentiate those of GABA result in increase of chloride flux and reduction in anxiety. Opposite actions that reduce GABA function increase anxiety.

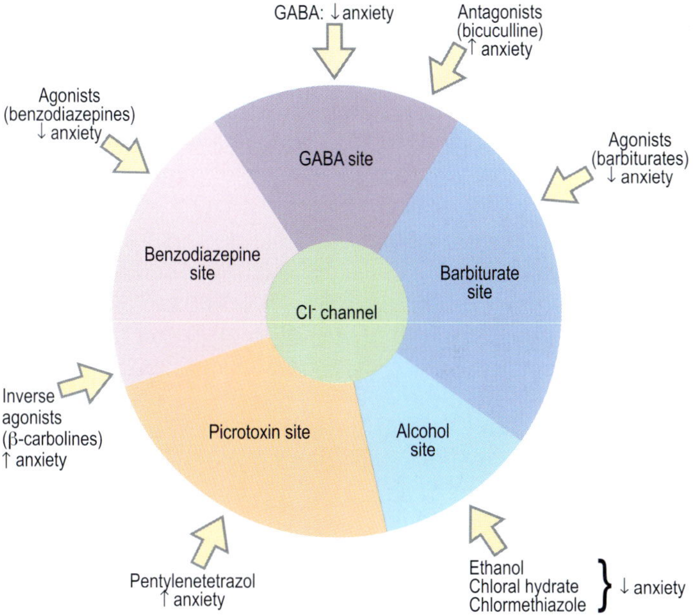

that the most likely explanation is decreased endogenous benzodiazepine agonism. It seems unlikely that this result is due to cerebral hypoperfusion.[72] An alternative explanation may be increased occupancy of the receptors by endogenous benzodiazepine inverse agonists such as β-carbolines.

Using fractal analysis, they also showed that regional benzodiazepine receptors of the left hemisphere in patients with GAD are more homogeneously distributed than in healthy subjects. Tiihonen et al[70] concluded that regional heterogeneity in blood perfusion, metabolism and receptor density is necessary to maintain the adaptability of the living organism, an ability that is lost in anxiety states.

Serotonin (5HT)

The neurons of this monoamine transmitter originate mainly in the dorsal and median raphe nuclei of the brainstem. Their axons diffusely supply the forebrain. Differences in the anatomy and pharmacology of these projections suggest both a specialization in function and a role in coordinating various brain functions, e.g. mood, sleep, impulse control, personality, psychosis etc. Deakin and Graeff[73] have suggested that two separate serotonergic pathways, originating from the dorsal raphe nucleus, are involved in anxiety. An ascending pathway to the amygdala and frontal cortex is thought to be involved in anticipatory anxiety and conditioned fear, therefore serving as a model for GAD. Another pathway, to the periaqueductal gray matter, is thought to mediate panic (unconditioned fear). A variety of pre- and postsynaptic 5HT receptors have been described (Figure 2). At least two of them, 5HT-1A and 5HT-2, have been implicated in GAD. Although 5HT almost certainly has a role in anxiety,[74] it is currently very difficult to specify whether the problem in GAD (as in other anxiety disorders) is an excess or a deficit of this transmitter. Furthermore, at present we cannot give a clear account of the mechanisms by which the serotonergic drugs produce their effects.

The levels of serotonin in the cerebrospinal fluid (CSF) appear to be lower in patients with GAD compared with controls.[75] Conversely, the activation of serotonin receptors by *m*-chlorophenylpiperazine (*m*-CPP) causes increased anxiety and anger-like responses in patients with generalized anxiety.[76]

Buspirone is an effective treatment for GAD (Chapter 8). It is a partial 5HT-1A agonist, and its effect could be achieved either through inhibiting release of serotonin by stimulating presynaptic autoreceptors or through promoting postsynaptic receptor function[63] (Figure 2). Serotonin reuptake inhibitors (SSRIs) block the reuptake of 5HT from the synaptic cleft back to the cell, thus increasing the availability of the transmitter to stimulate postsynaptic receptors (Figure 2).

Other subtypes of serotonin receptors, e.g. 5HT-2, seem to be involved in GAD. A number of antidepressants, e.g. amitriptyline and clomipramine, are antagonists of 5HT-2A receptors and they are useful anxiolytics (Chapter 6). 5HT-2C antagonists oppose the actions of *m*-CPP and may have anxiolytic properties. Further, long-term use of SSRIs and MAOIs desensitize this receptor and this may explain their effectiveness in anxiety.[74]

The involvement of serotonin in GAD is further supported by the genetic finding discussed earlier in this chapter, that a polymorphism of the gene regulating the serotonin transporter system accounts for a percentage of the anxiety-related personality traits.[62]

Noradrenaline (NA)

This catecholamine originates in the brain from cells located in a series of brainstem nuclei, mainly the locus coeruleus. These nuclei project to the whole of the forebrain. Noradrenaline is not only involved in arousal, attention and learning but also in emotional behaviour. Of the adrenergic receptors described (Figure 5), the a2 is the one linked with anxiety.

The plasma levels of catecholamines and their metabolite 3-methoxy-4-hydroxyphenylglycol (MHPG) in patients with GAD at rest, in most studies, are not different from those of controls.[77,78] Direct comparison with depression produced a graded profile of plasma noradrenaline levels.[79] The order of mean values was (from higher to lower): melancholic depression, non-melancholic depression, GAD, normal controls. Although only the values of the melancholic patients differed from the controls at a statistically significant level, the results provide some evidence for sympathetic overdrive in GAD.

Figure 5
Noradrenergic neuron and receptors. Presynaptic α_2 receptor is implicated in anxiety an postsynaptic β receptor mediates the autonomic symptoms associated with anxiety.

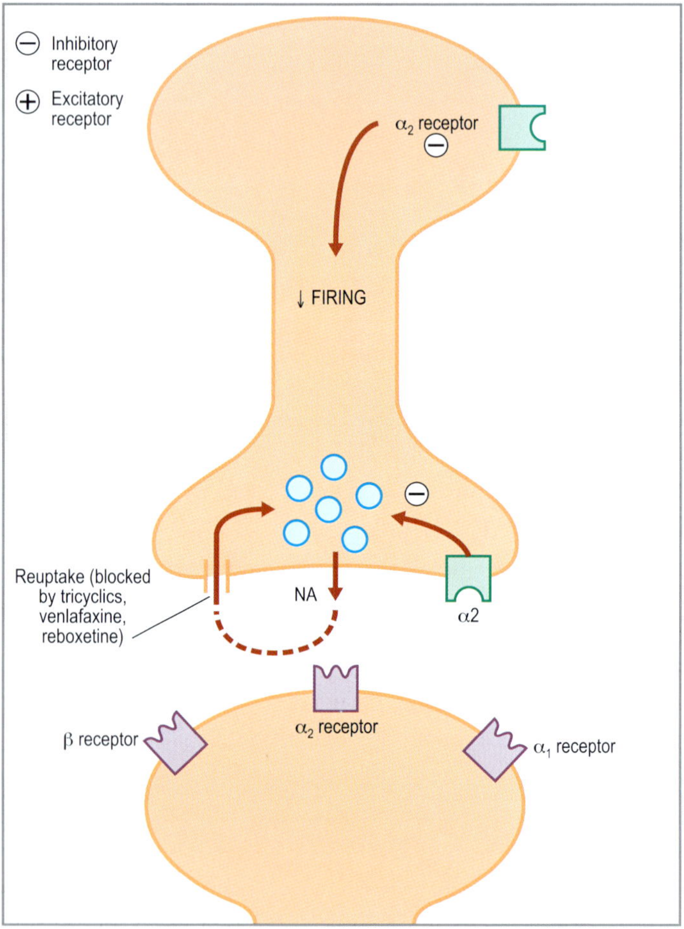

On the other hand, the levels of the enzymes responsible for the degradation of catecholamines, e.g. monoamine oxidase A (MAO-A) and catechol-*o*-methyl transferase (COMT) are not different from controls either.[80]

Challenge paradigms though show evidence of abnormality. Similar to depression and panic disorder, there is blunted growth hormone (GH) response to the a2 partial agonist clonidine in GAD patients. This finding suggests a postsynaptic a2 receptor hyposensitivity, which could be the result of chronic NA release. However, this may be due, at least partly, to abnormal GH feedback mechanisms.[81]

Cholecystokinin (CCK)

This peptide neurotransmitter is abundant in the brain, interacting extensively with GABA, 5HT and noradrenaline systems, and is thought to play a modulatory role in human anxiety. So far little specific evidence exists of its involvement in GAD. Injection of pentagastrin, an agonist of the type B receptor of cholecystokinin, in patients suffering from generalized anxiety induces panic attacks at higher rates than in controls though less than in panic disorder patients.[63]

Neuroendocrinology

The hypothalamic–pituitary–adrenal (HPA) axis links the brain with the rest of the body by means of its neuroendocrine function. The activation of this axis is an important component of the stress response of body and mind as a whole (Figure 6).

Unlike some forms of depression, the baseline plasma levels of corticotrophin releasing factor (CRF) and free cortisol, the end product of the axis, are not elevated in GAD patients compared with controls.[63,79] However, challenge paradigms of the integrity of the axis, such as the dexamethasone suppression test (DST), produce an irregular response in up to 38% of GAD patients. This suggests an abnormality in the regulatory mechanisms of the HPA axis, and abnormal stress responses in some GAD patients,[63] though in a lesser percentage than found in depressed patients.

Figure 6
The hypothalamic–pituitary–adrenal (HPA) axis in stress (simplified).

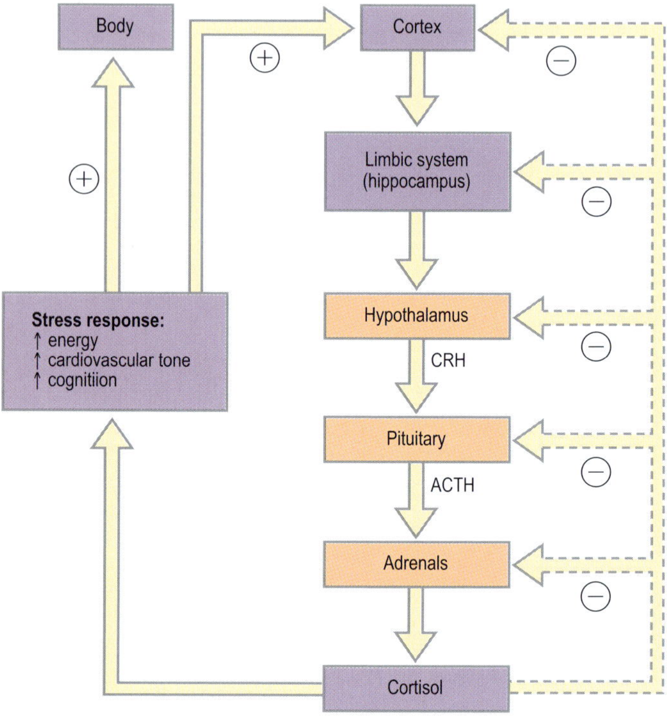

CRH: Corticotrophin-releasing hormone
ACTH: Adreno-corticotrophic hormone
+: Positive feedback
–: Negative feedback

Neurophysiology

The autonomic responses, such as electrodermal activity (measured by skin conductance), respiration, blood pressure and heart rate variability, when measured at rest, do not differ between GAD patients and controls.[82] In the same study, during stress tasks, patients with generalized anxiety showed significantly attenuated skin conductance, slower habituation and narrower range in heart rate (Table 11). These results indicate that sympathetic inhibition (instead of enhancement) occurs in GAD patients. These subjects may also be seen as having less 'autonomic flexibility', i.e. weaker autonomic responses to stress and more prolonged time to recovery than normal people.[63]

Exploring this idea further, Thayer et al[83] examined the autonomic characteristics of GAD and concluded that decreased cardiac vagal control discriminated GAD subjects and characterized the condition's distinguishing feature: worry. They revisited the list of most frequently endorsed subjective symptoms of generalized anxiety, and observed that several, including palpitations, being keyed up, restlessness, lack of concentration and sleep problems, may be associated with diminished parasympathetic function. They consider their view as compatible with the idea of reduced autonomic flexibility. However, they argue, the opposing notion of 'autonomic hyperactivity' should be excluded from the diagnostic criteria of GAD. They also reported that, in a pilot study, successful cognitive–behaviour therapy in a small sample of GAD patients appeared to increase vagal cardiac control.

Symptoms relating to motor tension, vigilance and scanning are frequently and reliably endorsed by GAD sufferers, as opposed to those of autonomic hyperactivity.[84] Increased muscle tension at rest has been reported[85] and it is thought to reflect heightened central nervous system arousal more accurately than do other peripheral physiological measures. The increased arousal is suggestive of the subject perceiving the environment as more threatening.

The electroencephalographic (EEG) data comparing GAD patients with non-anxious individuals at rest are equivocal. It is suggested that right hemispheric activity, thought to be involved in the processing of negative emotions and emotional stimuli in general, may be more strongly correlated with the increased peripheral muscular tone, thus facilitating the flight and escape behaviours associated with anxiety.[85] EEG mapping during the late morning hours demonstrated hypervigilance and increased sleep pressure, while in cognitive/psychophysiological tests, at the same time, critical flicker frequency, fine motor activity and reaction time were worsened.[86]

Subjective sleep quality in GAD is poor, and polysomnography shows difficulty in initiating and maintaining sleep, reduced slow wave sleep and reduced total sleep time and sleep efficiency.[87] Compared with depressed patients, no significant changes in REM latency or REM percentage of sleep time were observed. In fact, these last two measures seem to discriminate very well between the two diagnoses.[79] Therefore a vicious circle is established: hypervigilance and hyperarousal lead to nocturnal insomnia, which then causes diurnal tiredness.[86]

Summary

The neurobiological puzzle of GAD is still incomplete. However, on most measures studied in rest conditions, patients with generalized anxiety do not differ from normal controls, while their response to stressful stimuli are abnormal.[63] These abnormalities involve the NA, 5HT, GABA and CCK transmitter systems, as well as the HPA axis and some psychophysiological responses.

These findings appear to fit with Gray's neuroanatomical model for anxiety, which he labelled the 'behavioural inhibition system' (Figure 7).[88] According to this model the assessment of threat related stimuli (punishment, novelty, and non-presentation of expected reward) takes place in the septohippocampal area. The presence of threat activates the behavioural inhibition system and the result is increased arousal and suppression of the regular ongoing behaviours.

Figure 7
Gray's neuroanatomical model of generalized anxiety disorder (Behavioural Inhibition System).

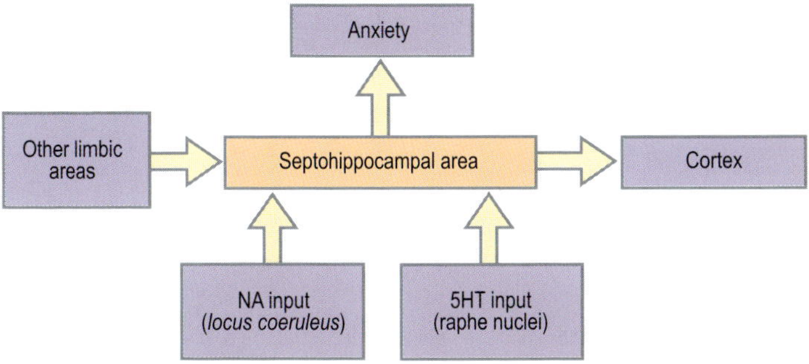

This state mimics persistent anxiety states, like GAD.[63] Serotonergic and noradrenergic input in the septohippocampal area further activates this system. It must be emphasised, however, that this theory is still tentative and a lot of research needs to be done in humans before any firm conclusions are drawn.

Psychosocial causes (Table 12)

Parenting

There has long been recognition that disturbed family relationships may be important in the development of anxiety disorders. Bowlby[89] proposed that a parent, or other attachment figure, functions to provide a secure base. Anxiety, in this model, reflects an insecure response to an actual or threatened separation from an attachment figure. Bowlby characterized dysfunctional parent–child relationships as being either 'disrupted' or 'distorted'.[90] Disruptions, that included such events as parental separation or death, though causing short-term distress, are not thought to be an impor-

Table 12
Psychological causes of GAD.

Parenting — low care, overprotection, affectionless	
Life events — dangerous or threatening events	
Cognitive process — attentional bias to threatening information	

tant factor in the development of serious long-term disturbance. Bowlby described a number of distortions to parenting. Firstly, the parent could be unresponsive to the child's needs. Secondly, the parent could be undermining, disparaging or rejecting of the child. Finally, the parent–child relationship could be inverted so that the child functioned to meet the parent's emotional needs. Current thinking,[91] which is consistent with this model, suggests that parenting can be described by two broad constructs: care and control, and overprotection.

A number of studies in adults have measured these dimensions using the Parental Bonding Instrument (PB1).[92] Their outcome[93] suggests that higher levels of anxiety are linked with reports of low parental care and with parental overprotection. Moreover, it was found that patients with anxiety neurosis were significantly more likely than controls to rate their parenting as less caring and more protective.[94] In addition, they were four times more likely to report their parenting as being characterized by affectionless control, the most pathological dimension. When this study was repeated using DSM-III-R criteria it confirmed the previous findings.[95] In particular those suffering with GAD showed a much greater chance of rating their parenting as aberrant, including affectionless control, where parenting is overprotective but neglectful.

This finding is supported by other work,[19] which followed a cohort of young adults through their third decade. In this study family problems were explored in retrospect. It was found that subjects with depression or anxiety (panic or GAD) or both were more likely than controls to report conflicts between parents, conflicts with parents, a lack of attention or care, and sexual trauma. Thus it would seem that, though inadequate parenting does seem to predispose to anxiety in general, and GAD in particular, it is not a specific relationship.

Life events and traumata

A number of studies have found that life events are important in the aetiology of GAD. Subjects with GAD were more likely than those with panic disorder to report an early parental death.[96] It was also found that GAD was more prevalent amongst those who had experienced an unexpected stressor.[97] A number of studies that have looked at the consequences of specific life events, such as rape or combat, have found that GAD is a common sequela.[98] These findings are consistent with a study of DSM-III-R GAD in which patients were compared with controls and were found to be significantly more likely to report exposure to a potentially traumatizing event.[99] Brown and Harris, who have studied this area extensively, conclude that like depressive illness, anxiety disorders, including GAD, are commonly provoked by a severe event during the six months preceding onset.[100] Moreover, it has been demonstrated that, while in depression, events associated with loss are more common, in anxiety disorders the association is with dangerous or threatening events. In contrast to depression, Brown et al[100] found that current social circumstances were not important in the aetiology of anxiety disorders. It is suggested that life events, particularly those associated with danger, have a causal role in the development of the core psychopathology of GAD: chronic anxious anticipation and constant perception of threat. Moreover, once GAD is established, traumatic events will function to maintain high levels of anxiety.[101]

Cognitive psychology

Beck and Emery[102] proposed that pathological anxiety derives from the misperception of danger that results from distortions in the way information is processed. Research is consistent in finding differences in the cognition and behaviour of those with GAD when compared with controls. For example, patients employ subtle avoidance in both motor behaviour[103] and cognitive activity.[104] Further, research using a Stroop paradigm found that there is an attentional bias to threatening or potentially threatening information.[105] The presence of such a cognitive bias was confirmed with a study which showed that GAD patients, compared with normal controls, exhibited increased vigilance for threatening facial expressions relative to neutral expressions. Therefore, the attentional bias operates for subtle non-verbal stimuli.[106] In addition, a number of studies have found autonomic inhibition and rigidity rather than sympathetic activation,[107] consistent with attempts to avoid threat and the effects of danger.

One reason for this may be that worry reduces somatic reactivity, and so functions to prevent emotional processing.[108] This lack of proper processing in turn contributes to the maintenance of anxious meanings and responses.[109] Finally, in GAD anxious subjects perceive themselves as having a lack of control over aversive stimuli. This functions to increase the aversive properties of those stimuli.[110]

Thus anxious cognitions interact with other processes to maintain the spiral of anxiety (Figure 8). Further evidence to support this view is provided by the fact that both cognitive therapy and cognitive behaviour therapy are effective in the treatment of GAD.[111]

An increasing number of studies is devoted to the process of pathological worry, central to the current concept of GAD, and the development of theoretical cognitive models that

Figure 8
The spiral of cognitively induced anxiety.

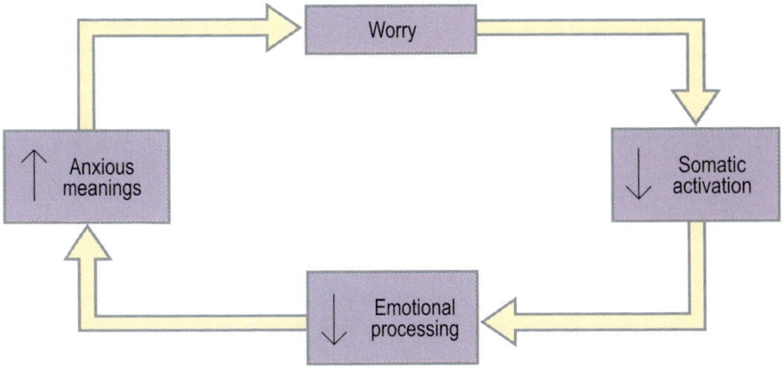

attempt to understand and explain it.[112] These models incorporate the evidence presented above, as well as some of the neurophysiological findings described earlier in this chapter. Worry, compared to other cognitive activity, is characterized by a reduction in present-oriented statements, increase in anxious and depressive affect, fewer shifts across topics, predominance of words that imply catastrophic interpretation (always, never, awful, terrible), and predominance of thoughts over images.[113] The latter is central to the model proposed by Borkovec and his colleagues.[114] Verbal thoughts elicit much smaller cardiovascular response compared with images of the same material. It is therefore hypothesized that the use of verbalization in the process of worry decreases autonomic arousal in response to threatening material, and this may account for the reduced autonomic reactivity seen in GAD. Worry is then negatively reinforced by the decrease in somatic symptoms, and develops into a secondary "worry about worry": if I worry the feared events will not happen.[115]

But what is the origin of the worry in the first place? One explanation derives from the observation that chronic worriers tend to doubt themselves and they catastrophize in terms of their perceived personal inadequacy in dealing with problems.[116] Although these worriers may not lack problem solving skills, but only the confidence to deal with matters as they arise, the non-occurrence or the successful negotiation of the feared event only helps to establish and reinforce the cognitive pattern of worrying. Another model[117] proposes the "intolerance of uncertainty" as a crucial factor in the development of worry. Research evidence is gradually accumulating for the models described here. Further, there is considerable overlap between them. It is, therefore, conceivable that a unifying cognitive conceptual model of pathological worry and GAD will emerge in the near future.

Depression and generalized anxiety

Depression and anxiety disorders are often found in the same patients (comorbidity). The epidemiological findings suggest a strong link between depression and generalized anxiety disorder in particular. In the National Comorbidity Survey in USA, 64.2% of patients with GAD have experienced at least one episode of depression in their lifetime.[17] Conversely, the same survey showed that 17.2% of depressed patients also had GAD. In fact, the odds ratio for major depression co-occurring with GAD was 6.0 (Table 13), higher than any of the other anxiety disorders.[118] When Goldberg investigated the relationship of anxiety and depressive symptoms in a large sample of community care attenders, he found a considerable overlap between the two, the correlation coefficient being 0.68. As for specific diagnosis, depression occurred in 4.9% of the sample, GAD in 3.9% and comorbidity of the two disorders in 2.1%.[119]

Despite their close inter-relationship and overlap in symptoms,[120] psychometric evidence suggests that anxiety and depression can be validly and reliably assessed separately (Figure 9). Physiological instability is associated with GAD, while apathy, retardation and withdrawal are more characteristic of depression. Patients with generalized anxiety also differ significantly from those with major depression on the

Table 13
Comorbidity of depression with other disorders (expressed as odds ratio, adapted from ref. 103).

Generalized anxiety disorder	6.0
Agoraphobia	3.4
Simple phobia	3.1
Social phobia	2.9
Panic disorder	4.0
Post-traumatic stress disorder	4.0
Alcohol dependence	2.0
Drug dependence	2.0
Dysthymia	2.8
Conduct disorder	1.3

Figure 9
Overlap and discrimination of anxiety and depressive symptoms.

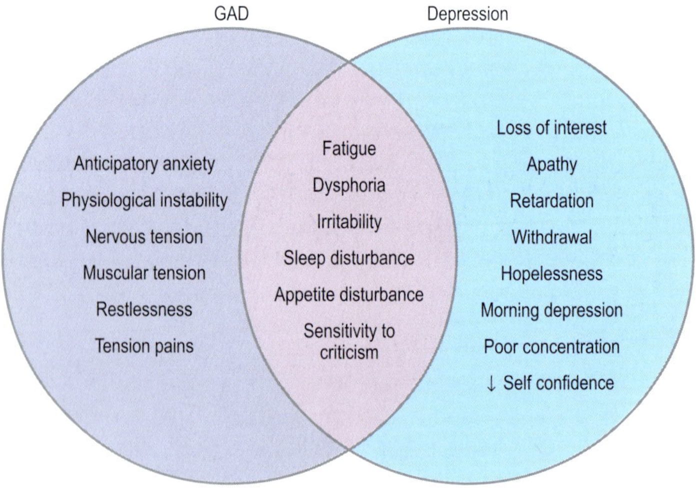

dimension of anticipatory and social anxiety. Further, latent trait analysis of Present State Examination symptoms identified two traits: a generalized anxiety trait, characterized by subjective nervous tension, muscular tension, tension pains, irritability, delayed sleep and restlessness, and a depression trait characterized by loss of interest, hopelessness, morning depression, inefficient thinking, poor concentration and lack of self-confidence.[121]

The relationship of GAD and depression is of great practical significance for the course and outcome of these conditions (Table 14). The anxiety disorder is more likely to precede the onset of the depressive illness. Individuals with depression secondary to GAD report more severe symptoms and greater social dysfunction, are twice as likely to seek medical advice and have a higher risk of hospitalization than patients with pure depression. Suicide is also more common in individuals with comorbid depression and anxiety. Patients with high anxiety ratings are slower to respond to treatment and recover from their episode of depression.[120,121]

Table 14
Impact of comorbid GAD on depression.

↑ Severity of depressive symptoms
↑ Social dysfunction
↑ Consultations
↑ Hospitalization
↑ Suicide risk
Slower & less complete response to treatment

This close relationship is also important in clarifying the nosological status of GAD. Three theoretical models are proposed in an attempt to explain the overlap between depression and anxiety (Figure 10). The first describes anxiety and depression as discrete disorders with clearly defined boundaries and diagnostic criteria as well as separate treatments. Patients can have either condition but not both of them at the same time. The second proposes that both conditions can occur at the same time. The third postulates that the co-occurrence of the two conditions represents a distinct entity, a mixed anxiety-depressive disorder. These models have been labelled traditional, comorbid and mixture/subsyndromal respectively.[121,122] They illustrate the debate on whether GAD deserves an independent diagnostic status or is better seen as an epiphenomenon of depression, even a personality disorder predisposing to affective illness.[120,121] In practice, the increased use of antidepressants in GAD makes such debate less critical for the average practitioner as these drugs treat both conditions.

Figure 10
Models of relationship of GAD with depression (order of occurrence may vary).

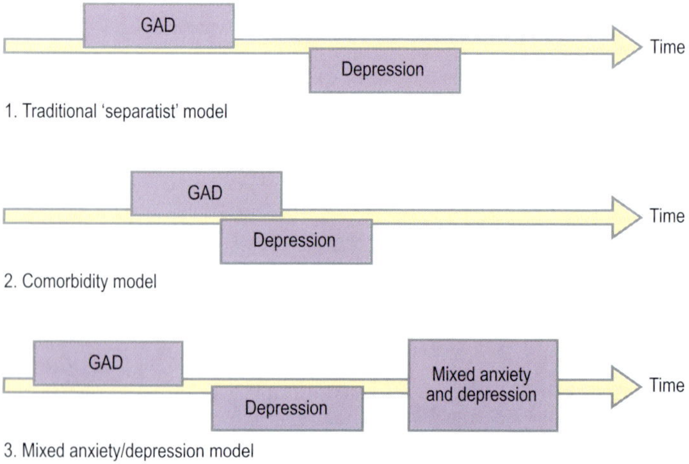

The two conditions are also genetically closely linked (Figure 11). Patients with comorbid depression and GAD have twice as many relatives with depression compared with patients suffering either depression or GAD alone.[121] Kendler, studying a large sample of female–female twins, concluded that major depression and GAD are the result of the same genetic factors but partly different environments. The genes that influence the liability to major depression also influence the liability to GAD and vice versa. While some environmental factors and life events appear to be both depressogenic and anxiogenic, precipitating mixed episodes of anxiety and depression, others are relatively specific in their impact. Life events related to exposure to danger appear to predispose to pure GAD, while events related to loss are more likely to result in pure depressive episodes.[120,123]

Figure 11
Genetic link of GAD with depression.

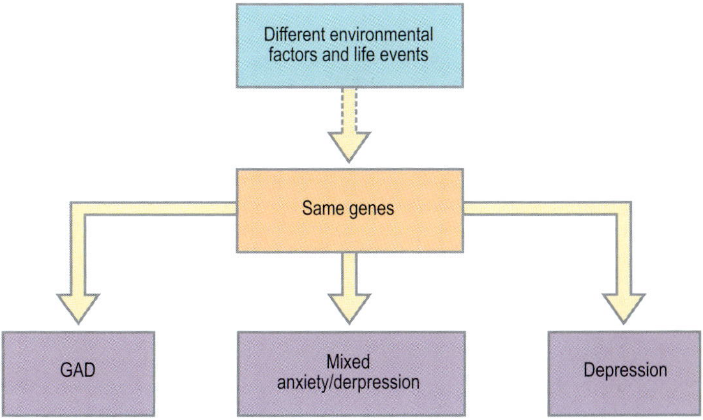

GAD and panic disorder

The separation of panic disorder from GAD in DSM-III was not without controversy for, following the tradition of Freud, many psychiatrists regarded panic attacks to be an index of severity of anxiety rather than a separate entity. For example, Marks wrote: 'the DSM-III-R elevated panic into an organising principle, yet it is no more diagnostic than the presence of anxiety'.[124] Furthermore, it was argued that the symptoms of panic are common to nearly all anxiety disorders as well as occurring in major depression. In addition, it has been found that a third of young adults had experienced panic in the preceding year, particularly those who experience high trait anxiety. Thus Tyrer commented: 'panic is a common station along the track to other neurotic destinations'.[125]

The phenomenology of panic

A panic attack is defined in DSM-IV[7] as a discrete period of intense fear or discomfort that is accompanied by at least 4 of 13 somatic or cognitive symptoms (Table 15). Where the attack is accompanied by less than 4 symptoms it is referred to as 'limited symptom attack'.

Table 15
Phenomenology of panic disorder (from DSM-IV).

Panic attacks
Discrete periods, with sudden onset, of intense apprehension, fearfulness or terror, often associated with feelings of impending doom.

Symptoms associated with panic attacks
1. Palpitations, pounding heart, or accelerated heart rate
2. Sweating
3. Trembling or shaking
4. Sensations of shortness of breath or smothering
5. Feeling of choking
6. Chest pain or discomfort
7. Nausea or abdominal distress
8. Feeling dizzy, unsteady, lightheaded or faint
9. Derealization (feelings of unreality) or depersonalization (being detached from oneself)
10. Fear of losing control or going crazy
11. Fear of dying
12. Paraesthesias (numbness or tingling sensations)
13. Chills or hot flashes

Panic can be either situational or spontaneous. Situational or cued panic arises in response to particular circumstances or cues. For example, an agoraphobic individual may panic when entering a supermarket, or when anticipating doing so. In some cases the cue is invariably linked to the onset of an attack, in which case it is classified as 'situationally predisposed panic'. In contrast, uncued, or non-situational, panic occurs without identifiable cues, and arises apparently spontaneously or 'out of the blue'. It is the nature of the second form of panic that is in dispute for, while some regard it to be on a continuum with generalized anxiety, others do not.

Panic disorder

The core feature of panic disorder is the presence of recurrent spontaneous panic attacks followed by at least 1 month of persistent concern about having further attacks.[7] The panic attacks in panic disorder are characterized by the absence of any situational trigger. The frequency of panic attacks is variable, and the presence of limited symptom attacks is common. Sufferers make characteristic attributions with respect to their panic attacks. Commonly, they are attributed to a life-threatening physical illness, particularly of cardiac origin. Alternatively, individuals may think that they are going mad or losing control. As sufferers are frequently very sensitive to physical symptoms, which are interpreted as having a potentially catastrophic outcome, they often present to GPs and specialists with concerns for their physical heath. The sensitivity to physical symptoms also complicates the treatment, for it leads to an intolerance of the side-effects of medication and means that the individual requires reassurance in order to comply with treatment. The main considerations in differential diagnosis are shown on Table 16.

Table 16
Differential diagnosis of panic disorder.

Anxiety due to medical condition (e.g., thyroid disease, anaemia)
Substance-induced anxiety
Depression
Social phobia
Specific phobias
Generalized anxiety disorder
Obsessive-compulsive disorder
Post-traumatic stress disorder
Delusional disorders

In common with GAD, panic disorder is accompanied by high levels of comorbidity, not only with other anxiety disorders but also with major depression and substance abuse. Major depression is found in 50%–65% of those with panic disorder, but in about one-third of these depression is found to precede the onset of panic. GAD occurs in about 25% of those with panic disorder. As currently defined, panic disorder has a life-time prevalence of 1.5%–3.5% and a 1 year prevalence of 1%–2%. In community samples, 30%–50% have associated agoraphobia. Generally, panic disorder begins between adolescence and the mid-30s, and tends to run a chronic course with its severity waxing and waning. For some the symptomatology is continuous and severe.[7]

The relationship between GAD and panic disorder

Given that panic disorder and GAD were considered a unitary disorder, 'anxiety neurosis', it is not surprising that the diagnostic boundaries between the two are in some respects blurred. Indeed, there is a body of evidence that suggests that for about 30%–60% of subjects GAD represents a prodromal phase of panic disorder.[126,127] Furthermore, it has been found that those with a prodrome of generalized anxiety were more likely to have a secondary diagnosis of alcoholism and depression. These findings perhaps support the notion that generalized anxiety and panic form part of a continuum of increasing severity. Elsewhere,[128] it has been found that GAD more commonly followed the onset of panic disorder, usually within 2 months (Figure 12). Where this was the case, the course of the panic disorder tended to be more chronic and unremitting. Indeed, it was found to have a less favourable outcome than where panic disorder was comorbid with depression. It should be noted that the phenomenon of anticipatory anxiety that patients experience between panic attacks is very similar to that of GAD but restricted in its focus.

Figure 12
Patterns of comorbidity of panic disorder and GAD.

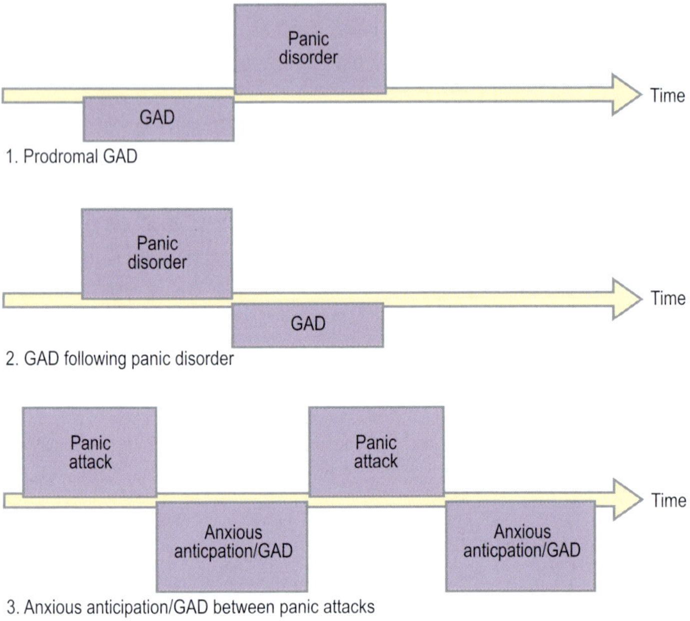

In spite of these findings, the bulk of evidence supports the separation of the two disorders. Firstly, family and twin studies support a distinction between them.[60] Two studies looking at first-degree relatives of probands with panic disorder with agoraphobia have found an increased incidence of panic disorder but not GAD.[129,130] Conversely, relatives of probands with GAD are found to have increased incidence of GAD but not panic disorder. In a twin study,[56] an increased incidence of anxiety disorders was found among monozygotic twins of panic and agoraphobia probands, as compared with dizygotic twins. There was no such difference between monozygotic and dizygotic twins of probands with GAD. This suggests that panic disorder is more influenced by genetic factors than is

GAD, where environmental factors may be more important. Secondly, a number of studies[131] have found that the onset of GAD tends to be both earlier and more gradual than that of panic disorder. While the former tends to begin in the early 20s, the latter has its onset in the mid-to late 20s.

The two disorders also differ in their symptom profiles.[131] GAD is characterized by symptoms of vigilance and scanning, including difficulty getting to sleep, poor concentration, an inability to relax and irritability (Table 17). Moreover, there is some evidence that this cluster of symptoms provides discriminant validity with respect to panic disorder. In contrast to panic disorder, those with GAD are seldom troubled by symptoms of autonomic hyperactivity. Again there are differences in the core cognitive components of the two disorders. GAD is characterized by the presence of excessive worry about life circumstances. The patients have cognitions related to interpersonal confrontation, competence, acceptance, concern about others and worry about trivia. On the other hand, panic disorder is dominated by threat-related cognitions and the tendency to misinterpret bodily symptoms as evidence of pending catastrophy.[132]

Finally, there is evidence of a distinction between the two disorders at a neurobiological level. In a study,[133] nine patients with panic disorder and nine with GAD underwent a 35% carbon dioxide challenge. It was found that, while both groups responded with an increase in autonomic symptoms, only those with panic disorder reacted with a large increase in subjective anxiety.

Thus panic disorder and GAD differ in many ways (Table 18), with panic disorder being dominated by autonomic hyperactivity and GAD being dominated by psychic anxiety. It is clear, therefore, that they do form two distinct disorders, albeit with a considerable comorbidity. Where there is comorbidity, the outcome is worse than for either disorder alone.

Table 17
The spectrum of panic and generalized anxiety symptoms (adapted from ref. 131).

Panic	Panic + GAD	GAD
Fear of dying/ going crazy	Nervousness/ apprehension	Restlessness
Trembling/shaking	Worry	Inability to relax
Dizziness	Muscle ache/ tension	Trouble getting to sleep
Lightheadedness	Fatiguability	
Breathlessness	Stomach distress	
Chest discomfort	Dry mouth	
Choking/ smothering	Tinnitus	
Something bad will happen imminently	Diarrhoea	
Palpitations	Blurred vision	
Numbness/tingling	Trouble swallowing	
Nausea/vomiting	Tendency to stutter	
Hold/cold spells	Irritability	
Sweating	Impatience	
	↓ Concentration	

Table 18
Summary of differences between panic disorder and GAD.

	Panic disorder	GAD
Genetic	↑ Genetic load influence	↑ Environmental
Age at onset	Late 20s	Early 20s
Symptoms	Autonomic hyperactivity	Vigilance/ scanning
Cognitive	Catastrophic interpretation of bodily symptoms	Excessive worry about life circumstances

GAD and obsessive-compulsive disorder

Obsessive-compulsive disorder (OCD) always stood out as a clearly defined, rather rare and circumscribed nosological entity, while the other anxiety disorders initially underwent a period of engagement to each other under the rubric of 'anxiety neurosis', and a subsequent divorce, but with some common ground having been eventually established in recent years. It was only after the advent of successful pharmacological and psychological treatments (i.e. clomipramine, SSRIs and cognitive–behaviour therapy), also effective in depression and other anxiety disorders, that the relationship between this condition and its neighbours became the focus of research. The publication of properly conducted epidemiological and genetic studies also dispelled the myth that OCD is rare, and generated a wealth of data regarding what is now referred to as OCD spectrum disorders, such as Tourette's syndrome (Table 19). These studies also evaluated the comorbidity of OCD with the rest of the depression–anxiety spectrum conditions.

Recent studies in the community reported a lifetime prevalence of 2.5% with a 1 year prevalence of 1.5%–2.1%. OCD is associated with depression and other anxiety disorders, as well as eating disorders. There is a high incidence of OCD in Tourette's syndrome (35%–50%), while a substantial number of OCD sufferers (20%–30%) have a history of tics.[7]

Table 19
The OCD spectrum disorders.

Obsessive-compulsive disorder
Tourette's syndrome
Body dysmorphic disorder
Trichotillomania
Pathological gambling

Phenomenology and diagnosis of OCD

OCD is characterized by the presence of recurrent obsessions and compulsions. Obsessions are ideas, thoughts, images or impulses that intrude upon the sufferer's consciousness and cause marked anxiety and distress; they are not simply excessive worries about real-life problems. Although they are recognized as the product of the person's own thought, they are experienced as alien and inappropriate, a quality also referred to as ego-dystonic. The most common obsessions relate to fears of being contaminated, repeated doubts about acts of the past, preoccupation with the perceived asymmetry of objects, aggressive or horrific impulses, and sexual imagery that contravene the person's moral beliefs. The individual usually tries to ignore or suppress the obsessions, or even neutralize them with a compulsion.

Compulsions are repetitive behaviours or mental acts that are not pleasureable but serve in preventing or reducing anxiety and distress, or even in preventing some dreaded event, often associated with an obsession. They are clearly excessive in their nature, and commonly involve washing and cleaning, mental counting and silent repeating of words, checking, repeating actions, asking for reassurance and ordering.

The disorder usually begins in adolescence for males and in early adulthood for females. In the majority of cases, the onset is insidious and, once established, OCD runs a chronic fluctuating course, with exacerbations often related to stress. The obsessions and compulsions are time consuming, and sufferers may spend hours every day engaging in them, to the detriment of their everyday life routines and occupational and social functioning.

Obsessions and compulsions may develop as part of anxiety disorder related to a general medical condition or substance abuse, in the course of a depressive episode or even a schizophrenic illness, and the exclusion of these conditions should be considered before a diagnosis is made.[7] The differential diagnosis is summarized in Table 20.

Table 20
Differential diagnosis of OCD.

Medical condition (e.g., encephalitis, Syndenham's chorea)
Substance-induced anxiety
Body dysmorphic disorder
Depression
Generalized anxiety disorder
Hypochondriasis
Specific or social phobia
Schizophrenia
Tic disorders
Eating disorders
Superstitions

The relationship between GAD and OCD

Evidence for a more subtle and intriguing relationship between these anxiety disorders comes from two different lines of research: quantitative genetics and psychopathology.

Black et al[134] studied the genetics of OCD, in relation to depression and GAD, in a blind, controlled fashion. They also attempted to look at the influence of comorbidity on their results. The prevalence rates of GAD and major depressive disorder were compared among first-degree relatives of subjects with OCD and comorbid GAD or major depression, respectively. It was found that the rates of depression were not increased in the relatives of the probands with comorbid OCD and depression. Rates of GAD in relatives of subjects with comorbid OCD and GAD were not increased either. However, the rates of GAD were increased in the relatives of the OCD probands, compared to the relatives of healthy controls. Although the authors treat their results with great caution, particularly because of the small sample size, they argue that, as in the case of Tourette's syndrome, GAD may represent an alternative expression of the genetic factors responsible for OCD. This adds to the argument for the existence of a 'general neurotic syndrome', in which the clinical expression of a genotype may differ among the carriers, thus producing a spectrum of effects.[135]

In DSM-IV,[7] the differential diagnosis of OCD and GAD is partly based on the distinction between obsessions and worries. The authors consider that the content of the former does not typically involve real-life problems, and the obsessions are experienced as inappropriate by the individual. On the other hand, it is thought that the person experiences worries as excessive concerns about real-life circumstances. This view is not universally supported by research on the psychopathology of worry. Investigations on the content of worry, and the differences in focus between the pathological worry that characterizes GAD and normal worry, show that GAD sufferers worry about things that normal people do not find problematic at all, e.g., minor, routine, daily hassles. On the other hand, GAD subjects distinguished themselves by having fewer worries related to work and school situations, areas that offer more circumscribed, problem focused and realistic worries.[136] Furthermore, the question 'Do you worry about minor things?' differentiated the GAD group of patients better than any other question. The authors call for more research into the realistic or unrealistic nature of specific worries.

It has been reported that patients with GAD score higher on the Maudsley Obsessional-Compulsive Inventory than do other clinically anxious groups.[137] The observation that worry and obsessional phenomena share a number of common features, i.e. both are repetitive and difficult to control, led to the more systematic exploration of the relationship between them.[138] A significant correlation was found between worry and checking and doubting but not washing or obsessional slowness. The authors observed that there is a functional similarity of worry and checking, in that they are both orientated towards a future threat. They suggested that GAD may represent a cognitive variant of obsessional checking. The relationship between worry and obsessive phenomena is summarized in Figure 13.

Figure 13
Relationship between obsessive-compulsive phenomena and worries.

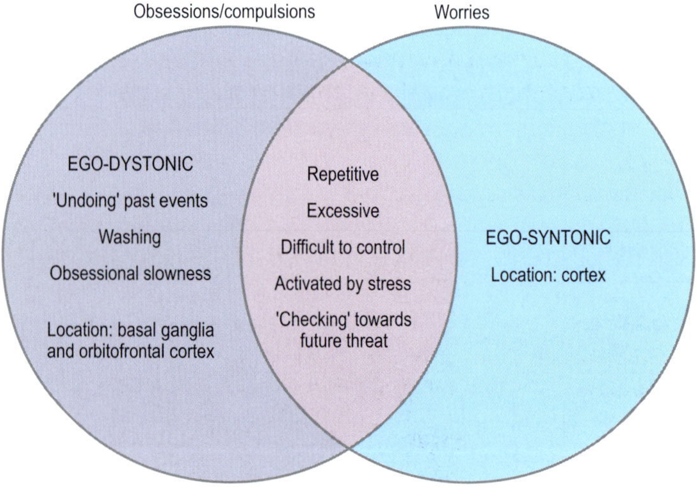

Treatment

Pharmacological treatments of GAD

A number of pharmacological agents from different classes of drugs have proved to be effective in the treatment of GAD (Table 21). As the neurobiology of the condition is becoming clearer, new and more specific agents are currently under investigation.

Benzodiazepines

Benzodiazepines have been the gold standard in the treatment of GAD for many years. They offer a rapid onset of action, with maximum effect achieved within 2 weeks. They

Table 21
Effectiveness of drug classes in GAD.

First line	Second line	Not effective
Venlafaxine SSRIs (Paroxetine) Buspirone TCAs Benzodiazepines	Flupenthixol (low dose) Hydroxyzine MAOIs	Beta-blockers

promote sleep and are generally well tolerated, although their sedating, muscle relaxing and amnesic properties may be problematic. It should also be remembered that the benzodiazepines potentiate the effect of alcohol, the most commonly used lay remedy to alleviate anxiety. Combined use can result in behavioural disinhibition and dangerously impaired psychomotor performance, e.g. in driving.

Diazepam has been the favourite in this class of drugs. Initiation of treatment with a small dose, e.g. 2 mg three times a day or 5 mg twice a day, allows tolerance to the psychomotor and sedative effects to develop, although higher doses (up to 30 mg/day of diazepam or equivalent) are usually needed.[139] The general recommendation for benzodiazepines is for a short course only. In practice many patients need them for much longer and this is justified if other options, such as buspirone and antidepressants, have failed.

Patients and clinicians are greatly concerned about the propensity of benzodiazepines to develop tolerance, physical dependence and withdrawal reaction on discontinuation. Rickels and his colleagues have extensively studied these phenomena. They found no evidence of dose escalation in patients with a mean time of 8 years of benzodiazepine use.[140] On abrupt discontinuation almost all of the patients suffered some withdrawal symptoms and a substantial proportion (up to 25%) were unable to stay off the drug eventually.[141] The withdrawal reaction occurred less frequently and was milder when the medication was gradually tapered or the patients were on long half-life rather than short half-life benzodiazepines.[142]

Buspirone

Buspirone, a partial 5HT-1a agonist, is effective in GAD, although the improvement is not apparent until 2–3 weeks into treatment. It is well tolerated and doesn't interact with alcohol. It may cause insomnia rather than sedation and it is not associated with tolerance, dependence or withdrawal. It is given in two or three divided doses, starting with 10–15 mg/day and gradually increasing up to 60 mg/day according to response.

Buspirone cannot alleviate the withdrawal symptoms of the benzodiazepines and it was initially thought that it is less effective in patients previously exposed to the latter class of drugs, possibly because of the lack of sedative effect.[143] More recent data indicate that this can be rectified if buspirone is started 2–3 weeks before the gradual withdrawal of the benzodiazepine.[144]

Tricyclic antidepressants (TCAs)

Some studies have shown that TCAs, especially imipramine, are effective in GAD. Kahn et al (1986) compared imipramine with chlordiazepoxide and demonstrated that, despite the good early response produced by the latter, at the end of the trial imipramine was slightly better in global efficacy with significantly better results in the feelings of tension and depressed mood.[145]

In another study,[146] 73% of patients showed marked or moderate improvement with imipramine compared with 69% on trazodone, 66% on diazepam and 47% on placebo. Patients with affective disorders were excluded so the results cannot be attributed solely to the treatment of underlying depression. More important, the initial worsening of symptoms that occurs when antidepressants are used in panic disorder (see Figure 14) did not happen with the GAD patients. The effective doses are comparable with the ones used in depression.

Venlafaxine

A growing body of evidence shows that venlafaxine, a serotonin and noradrenaline reuptake inhibitor (SNRI)

Figure 14
Time course of anxiolytic treatments in GAD.

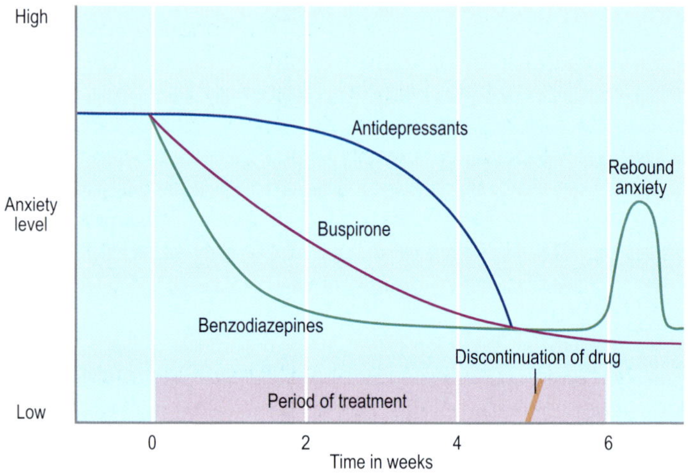

antidepressant, is effective in GAD. Initially, a meta-analysis of depression studies showed that venlafaxine, compared with placebo, produced significantly greater improvement in anxiety symptoms associated with depression.[147] Following this observation, the extended release preparation of the drug was tested in DSM-IV GAD populations without concomitant depression.

Efficacy and safety of venlafaxine in GAD was evaluated in a large (over 300 patients), double-blind, placebo-controlled, 8 week study.[148] The dose of the drug was fixed (75, 150 or 225 mg/day). The patients receiving medication showed a significantly better outcome than placebo in a range of outcome measures. The improvement was seen as early as the first week of the trial and persisted throughout the 8 weeks. Although all three venlafaxine doses demonstrated efficacy, this was more robust with the higher dose ie 225 mg/day. The medication was generally well tolerated. The majority of side effects, such as nausea, insomnia, dry mouth and dizziness, were mild to moderate, appeared early in the course of the study, and tended to subside as the treatment progressed.

Another double blind, 8 week study[149] compared venlafaxine with buspirone and placebo in outpatients with GAD. The maximum dose of venlafaxine in this study was 150 mg/day, while that of buspirone was 30 mg/day. Both drugs were superior to placebo, but venlafaxine showed an earlier effect. Further, venlafaxine showed advantage over buspirone in secondary outcome measures, notably the Hamilton Depression (HAD) scale anxiety subscore. Again, the medication was well tolerated and the adverse events were not different between groups.

Finally, the first long-term (6 months) trial of venlafaxine versus placebo (Figure 15) has recently been reported.[150] Compared with placebo, venlafaxine significantly improved anxiety on all primary outcome measures, from week 1 or 2 of treatment to the end of the study. At 6 months, the response rate for the venlafaxine group was 69% compared with 42% for the placebo group. In effect, this is the first study demonstrating the efficacy of any drug in the long-term treatment of GAD using the current diagnostic criteria for this condition. Based on the data from these trials, venlafaxine has recently been licensed for the treatment of GAD in a number of countries (Table 21).

An important finding that emerges from the studies comparing antidepressants and buspirone with benzodiazepines in GAD is that the antidepressants are better in treating the psychological symptoms of anxiety while the benzodiazepines appear superior in treating the somatic symptoms.

Selective serotonin reuptake inhibitors (SSRIs)

There is now published data on one SSRI (paroxetine) in the treatment of GAD, in a randomized, double-blind, placebo-controlled study of 324 patients over 8 weeks. Despite the

Figure 15
Venlafaxine versus placebo in GAD. Data from a 6 month study (ref. 150).

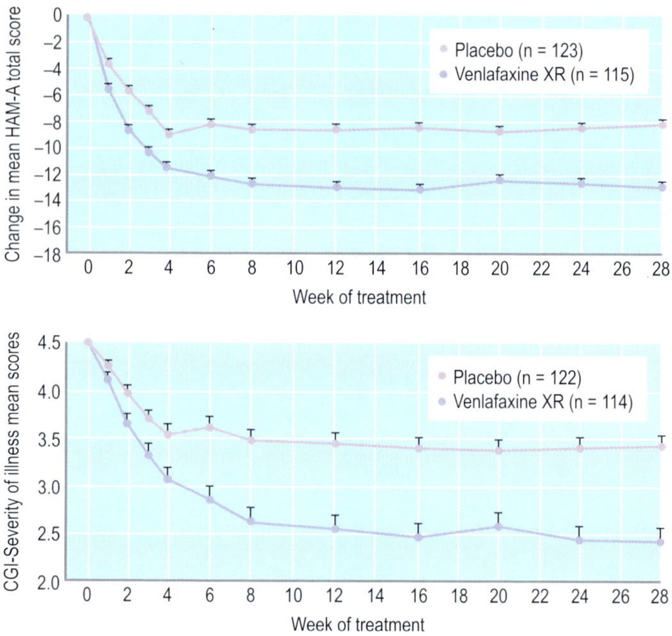

high placebo response (55.6%), the medication proved significantly superior, producing a response rate of 72.4% in the patients who completed the study. In some key symptom areas, such as anxious mood, significant difference over the placebo was seen as early as the first week of treatment, and was maintained throughout the study. Remission was achieved by over 42.5% of the patients that completed the trial, a result significantly better than the one observed with placebo (26.3%). The medication was generally well tolerated and the mean dose used was 26.8 mg/day.[151] Some evidence suggesting that paroxetine is also effective in relapse prevention has just been reported.[152] Despite the relative lack of randomized controlled trials, it is reasonable to predict that other SSRIs will also prove useful in this anxiety disorder (Table 22).

Table 22

Comparison of benzodiazepines, buspirone and antidepressants in the treatment of GAD.

	Benzodiazepines	Buspirone	TCAs	Venlafaxine/ paroxetine
Onset	Fast	Slow	Slow	Slow
Exacerbation	–	–	+/–	+/–
Therapeutic tolerance	Little	No	No	No
Withdrawal	++	–	+	+
Abuse	+	–	–	–
Interactions/ethanol	+++	+	+	+
Sedation	++	–	++	–
Amnesia	++	–	+	–
Overdose risks	–	–	++	–

Monoamine oxidase inhibitors (MAOIs and RIMAs)

Their use has not been properly evaluated in GAD. In the 1960s they were used to treat anxiety states in a non-specific way and, since they are effective in panic disorder and social phobia, it is reasonable to assume that they may be of value in GAD as well. The introduction in recent years of reversible inhibitors of monoamine oxidase, the RIMAs, such as moclobemide, which has a safe side effect profile compared with the old MAOIs, may lead to the re-evaluation of this class of drugs in generalized anxiety.

Antipsychotics

One antipsychotic (flupenthixol in low doses, e.g. 1–3 mg/day) is licensed for the treatment of depression and, as its name suggests, is also used to treat anxiety. In addition, low doses of other neuroleptics are sometimes used for the treatment of anxiety, e.g. thioridazine 25–50 mg two or three times a day. They are not as effective as benzodiazepines[153] and there is always the risk of akathisia with acute administration or of tardive dyskinesia with chronic use.

In recent years the use of depot injection (fluspirilene 1.5 mg weekly) has been studied. The drug demonstrated anxiolytic properties and was in general well tolerated but there was a very close positive relationship between tolerability and clinical outcome.[154]

Table 23
Selective Serotonin Reuptake Inhibitors (SSRIs) and their dose range (mg/day)

Citalopram	20–40
Fluoxetine	20–40
Fluvoxamine	50–200
Paroxetine	20–50
Sertraline	50–200

Overall, the available information to support the short-term use of antipsychotic drugs in GAD is very limited and in the case of long-term use almost non-existent. Further, no serious benefit/risk analysis has been undertaken so far.[155]

Hydroxyzine

This antihistamine (H1 blocker) drug acts rapidly as an anxiolytic even at doses as low as 50 mg/day.[156] At this level of dosing it is well tolerated without causing too much daytime sedation. It appears then to be a useful alternative in the treatment of generalized anxiety.

Beta-blockers

These drugs are firm favourites among general practitioners but there is very little evidence to justify their use in anxiety disorders. They are effective in controlling the peripheral noradrenaline-mediated symptoms of anxiety but this is not reflected in the psychological symptoms at all. In fact, patients may find the bradycardia resulting from the beta-blockers even more alarming and anxiety provoking.[139] They are dangerous in asthmatics and can cause depression. They should only be used when clearly indicated, e.g. to reduce performance anxiety in artists, especially musicians.

Treatment of GAD with comorbid depression, panic disorder and OCD

When depression is comorbid with GAD, the treatment of choice, for both conditions, is obviously an antidepressant. The presence of GAD should direct the clinician in choosing a compound that is effective in both conditions, mainly an SSRI or venlafaxine.

The first-line treatment of panic disorder has changed in recent years, moving from benzodiazepines to SSRIs. Studies with all the available drugs from this class (Table 23) have shown efficacy in panic disorder.[157] The lack of abuse potential, combined with the favourable side effect profile, makes them the treatment of choice for panic disorder with or without comorbid GAD. However, it should be remembered that, unlike GAD, panic symptoms may worsen during the first week of treatment with an SSRI.

In a similar fashion, there is now a substantial number of controlled studies showing that the compounds that act by blocking the reuptake of serotonin, clomipramine and the SSRIs, constitute the most effective pharmacological treatment of OCD.[158] It is reasonable then to choose from these drugs in the cases of comorbid OCD and GAD.

Future anxiolytic drugs

A number of novel drugs interacting with the benzodiazepine receptor complex, various serotonin receptor subtypes and neuropeptide receptors are undergoing clinical trials at present.[159] Some randomized controlled trials have already reported. The results appear to be positive for abecarnil, a partial benzodiazepine agonist.[160] Gepirone, a partial 5HT-1a agonist,[161] and serazepine, a 5HT-2 antagonist,[162] also show some positive results, while the picture with ondansetron, a 5HT-3 antagonist,[163] is still unclear. Finally, the results of cholecystokinin-B receptor antagonists are disappointing so far.[164]

Length of treatment

Given that GAD has a relatively early age of onset and tends to run a chronic course it seems reasonable that long-term treatment and maintenance may be required. Further, the relapse rate of the illness following acute treatment appears to be high.[165] Unfortunately, very little research has been conducted on the long-term management of the condition and many questions such as what is the difference between various drugs in tolerability, risks and efficacy in ongoing treatment, what the optimal dose is for maintenance and continuation therapy, and what the optimal length of treatment is following recovery, remain largely unanswered.[45] Indeed, we don't even know whether treatment after the acute episode alters the history of the illness or not. Until this information becomes available, it is safer and clinically justified to advise treatment for at least 6 months to 1 year after recovery, as with depression.

Predictors of outcome

Acute onset of illness, early intervention and positive response to previous treatment are good predictors. Compliance and realistic expectations from the treatment, good ego strength and martial stability also favour good outcome. The most important negative predictor is co-current personality disorder.[166]

Treatment resistant GAD

Unlike depression, the concept of treatment resistant anxiety disorders is not established and researched properly yet. We have no reliable data concerning the percentage of GAD patients who fail to respond to trials of medication given in adequate doses and for long enough to expect them to have an effect.

In assessing such a patient, it is reasonable to inquire about compliance, reconsider the diagnosis, look for comorbid conditions such as depression, alcohol and substance misuse, other anxiety disorders, personality disorders or medical illnesses and check for psychosocial factors that may impede progress.[167]

A rational approach then would be to switch to another class of drugs and give the maximum dose or, if this fails, to use a safe combination from two different classes (see algorithm, Figure 16). However, it must be emphasized that, unlike depression where lithium, buspirone, thyroid hormones etc. have been shown to enhance the action of antidepressants, augmentation strategies in GAD have not been tested formally yet.

Psychological treatment of GAD

Outcome studies

A number of psychotherapeutic interventions have been employed in the treatment of GAD. Where outcome studies have been conducted, it has been found that these interventions are significantly better at reducing symptoms than control conditions, e.g. where patients are monitored on a waiting list (Figure 17).[168,169] Therapies used include relaxation training, biofeedback, non-directive psychotherapy, behaviour therapy and cognitive therapy. Generally improvement is moderate, but it is found to be maintained at follow-up.[170] On average there is a reduction of approximately 50% in somatic symptoms as measured by the Hamilton Anxiety Scale (HAS) and a reduction of approximately 25% in the tendency to worry as measured by the Spielberger State-Trait Anxiety Inventory (STAI-T).

Barlow,[170] also provided an estimate of overall efficacy of benzodiazepines versus CBT. In his review, benzodiazepine-treated patients from the medication arms of 13 trials had an average 47.5% improvement in their HAS score compared with 30% for the placebo arms. He compares this with an average 54% improvement seen with psychotherapy. However, this form of analysis is somewhat deceptive. The

Figure 16
Algorithm for the pharmacological treatment of GAD.

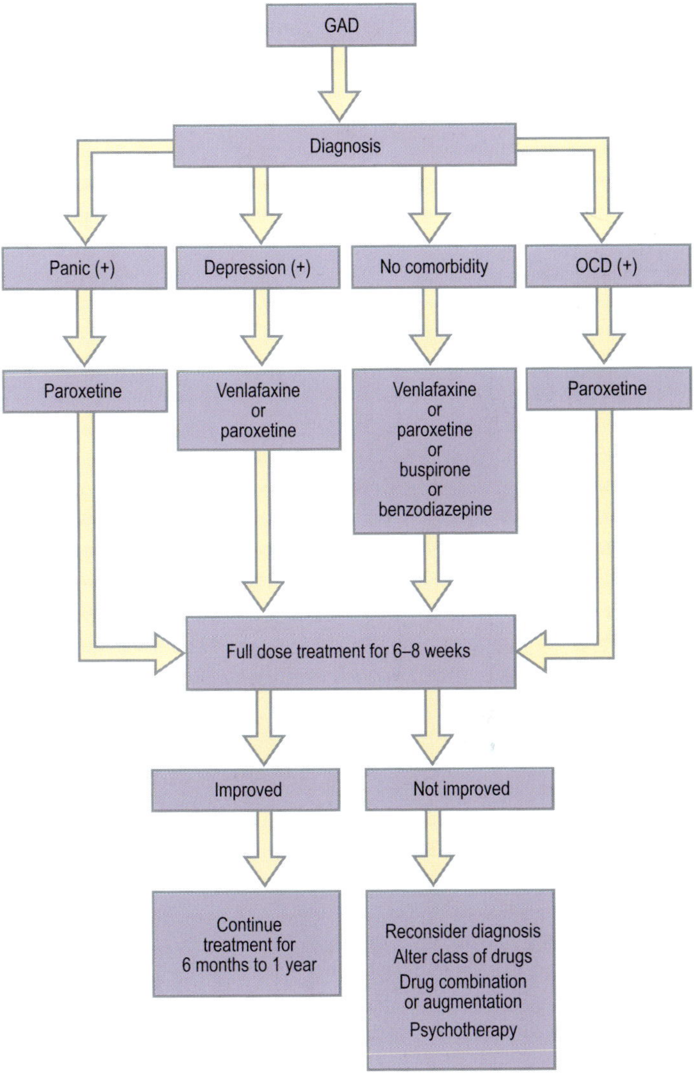

Figure 17
Comparative outcome from psychotherapeutic treatments in GAD (adapted from ref.[168]).

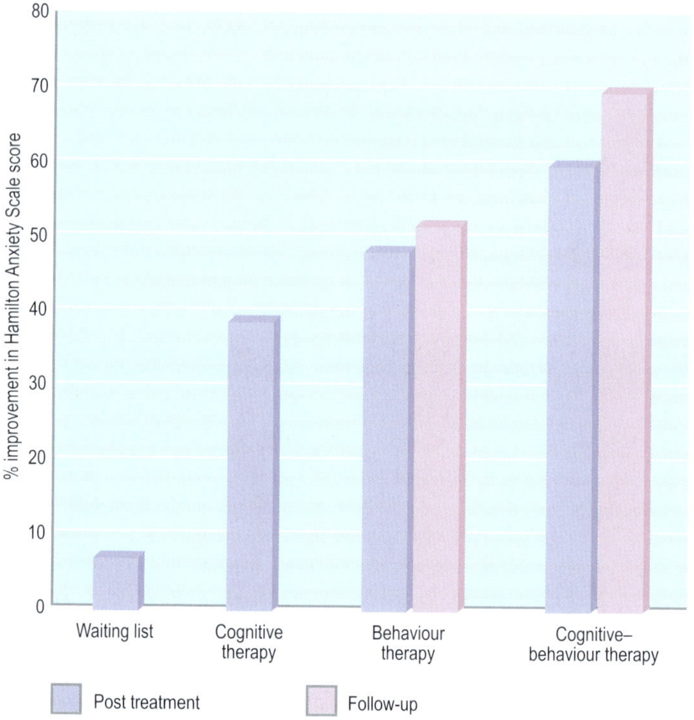

sample size in the psychotherapy studies is usually very small, averaging only 17 patients per group in the 11 studies performed since 1980.[111] Further, the 54% average reduction in HAS mentioned above represents the simple mean of all available results, without weighting for the different sizes of the trials. The largest study, with 24 patients, showed only 39% improvement, while the biggest improvement in HAS (76%) was seen in the smallest study (10 patients).

Where different modes of psychological treatment have been compared, Cognitive Therapy (CT) and Cognitive–Behaviour

Therapy (CBT) are generally found to produce the greatest symptomatic improvement. For example, in a study comparing CT with analytic psychotherapy and anxiety management in patients with GAD,[171] it was found that symptomatic improvement was greater with CT. At six month follow-up CT and anxiety management were superior to analytic psychotherapy. Importantly, patients rated themselves significantly more improved with CT than with other modes of treatment. At six month follow-up, about 60% of patients were considered to have achieved normative functioning with CT, as compared with 20% for analytic psychotherapy.

These findings are consistent with research which compared CBT, applied relaxation and non-directive therapy.[172] Results showed that applied relaxation and CBT were clearly superior to non-directive therapy. The improvements achieved in relaxation and CBT were maintained at twelve month follow-up. Where behaviour therapy and cognitive therapy have been compared[173] both achieved marked reactions in symptoms, and did not differ significantly from one another. When subjects were followed up, those who had received cognitive therapy appeared to have maintained their improvement better than those treated with behaviour therapy. Furthermore, while only 22% of patients achieved normative functioning with behaviour therapy, 57% of those receiving cognitive therapy were in the normative range at the end of treatment.[174]

When psychological treatment was compared with benzodiazepine medication,[175] it was found that the group taking medication showed the most immediate improvement. As treatment progressed the improvement diminished and by the end of the trial it was rated as minimal. The psychological treatment groups, who received either CBT or anxiety management training, continued to improve during the trial. At the trial's conclusion both showed consistent and significant change. At follow-up, CBT showed greatest improvement but the difference from anxiety management was not statistically significant.

A 10-week study[176] compared diazepam with CBT and the combination of the psychological treatment with the medication or placebo. The results of this trial suggested that diazepam plus CBT was more effective than CBT alone. However, the design of this study was far from ideal. The study had a small sample size (15 to 20 patients per group), the dose of diazepam used was too small, and the medication was tapered to zero after the 6th week of treatment.

Comparisons of CBT with venlafaxine and other antidepressants have not yet been conducted. It may prove a beneficial strategy to combine CBT with antidepressants, resulting in synergistic interaction between the two treatments.

In general, the evidence points to cognitive–behaviour therapy achieving clinically meaningful improvement at the end of treatment. The improvement is maintained at follow-up and in some instances further improvement has been reported. CBT is also associated with low drop-out rates and reduction in the use of medication.[177] However, serious methodological shortcomings, such as small sample sizes and unsatisfactory placebo conditions, undermine the rigour of the evidence. Further, properly trained therapists are still in short supply, especially in the National Health Service. This is a very important aspect of the delivery of CBT, since it has been shown that better trained therapists provide a more effective treatment.[178] On the positive side, the chronicity of untreated GAD and the absence of improvement in those maintained on a waiting list do suggest that good outcome with psychotherapy is not simply the result of spontaneous remission.

Factors affecting outcome in psychological treatments

While research suggests that psychological treatment does result in a significant improvement overall, it is found that some patients receive greater benefit than others (Table 24). It is observed that good outcomes in research are associated with samples that are free from benzodiazepines.[170] Though this might imply that anxiolytic medication functions to hinder psychological treatment, there are other interpretations. It may be that those taking medication have more severe illness. It is also likely that selection criteria which require patients to be off medication at the start of a trial, bias the sample to a group which is predisposed and responsive to a psychological approach. Certainly, previous treatment, whether psychological or medical, is found to relate to poorer outcome.[173,177] In this case it is likely that previous treatment is an indicator of greater severity. There is also a strong link between severity and duration of symptoms. In a study of GAD in over 350 women[22] it was found that those with longstanding illness had more symptoms which were of greater severity. Chronicity also results in a poorer outcome because it causes a negative expectation of change,[171] with a concomitant reduction in effort to learn new coping strategies, while existing maladaptive coping strategies are more entrenched. This has proved to be the case in all major psychiatric conditions, thus emphasizing the need for effective interventions that are established as early as possible, Finally, it is found that both those with psychiatric comorbidity and those with a coexisting personality disorder tend to be less responsive to psychological treatment.[170–179]

Table 24
Indicators of poor response to psychological treatment.

Previous treatment (psychological or pharmacological)
Concurrent medication
Longer duration of symptoms
Comorbid psychiatric illness
Coexisting personality disorder

References

1. Berrios GE, Link C. Anxiety disorders: clinical section. In: Berrios GE, Porter R, eds. *A History of Clinical Psychiatry.* London: Athlone Press, 1995.

2. Freud S. *The justification for detaching from neurasthenia a particular syndrome: the anxiety neurosis.* Collected papers, vol. 1, 76–106. London: Hogarth Press, 1953. Originally published in 1894.

3. Klein DF. Delineation of two drug-responsive anxiety syndromes. *Psychopharmacologia* 1964; **5**: 397–408.

4. Clark MJ. Anxiety disorders: social section. In Berrios GE, Porter R, eds. *A History of Clinical Psychiatry*. London: Athlone Press, 1995.

5. American Psychiatric Association (1980). Diagnostic and Statistical Manual of Mental Disorders, 3rd ed. (DSM-III). Washington, DC: American Psychiatric Association.

6. American Psychiatric Association (1987). Diagnostic and Statistical Manual of Mental Disorders, 3rd ed. (DSM-III-R). Washington, DC: American Psychiatric Association.

7. American Psychiatric Association (1994). Diagnostic and Statistical Manual of Mental Disorders, 4th ed. (DSM-IV). Washington, DC: American Psychiatric Association.

8. World Health Organisation (1992). The ICD-10 Classification of Mental and Behavioural Disorders. Geneva: World Health Organisation.

9. Anderson DJ, Noyes R Jr, Crowe RR. A comparison of panic disorder and generalized anxiety disorder. *Am J Psychiatry* 1984; **141**: 572–575.

10. Logue MB, Thomas AM, Barbee JG et al. Generalized anxiety disorder patients seek evaluation for cardiological symptoms at the same frequency as patients with panic disorder. *J Psychiatr Res* 1993; **27**: 55–59.

11. Wulsin LR, Arnold ML, Hillard JR. Axis I disorders in E.R. patients with atypical chest pain. *Int J Psychiatry Med* 1991; **21**: 37–46

12. Kane FJ, Harper RG, Wittels E. Angina as a symptom of psychiatric illness. *South Med J* 1988; **81**: 1412–16.

13. Carter CS, Maddock RJ. Chest pain in generalized anxiety disorder. *Int J Psychiatry Med* 1992; **22**: 291–98.

14. de Ruiter C, Garssen B, Rijken H et al. The hyperventilation syndrome in panic disorder, agoraphobia, and generalized anxiety disorder. *Behav Res Ther* 1989; **27**: 447–52.

15. Rapee R. Differential response to hyperventilation in panic disorder and generalized anxiety disorder. *J Abnorm Psychol* 1986; **95**: 24–28.

16. Blazer DG, Hughes D, George LK et al. Generalized anxiety disorder. In: Robins LN, Regier D, eds. *Psychiatric Disorders in America: The Epidemiologic Catchment Area Study*. New York, NY: The Free Press, 1991: 180–203.

17. Wittchen H-U, Zhao S, Kessler RC et al. DSM-III-R Generalized anxiety disorder in the National Comorbidity Survey. *Arch Gen Psychiatry* 1994; **51**: 355–64

18. Surtees PG, Dean C, Ingham JG et al. Psychiatric disorder in women from an Edinburgh community: Associations with demographic factors. *Br J Psychiatry* 1983; **142**: 238–46.

19. Angst J, Vollrath M. The natural history of anxiety disorders. *Acta Psychiatr Scand* 1991; **84**: 446–52.

20. Nystroem S, Lindergard B. Predisposition for mental syndromes: a study comparing predisposition for depression, neurasthenia and anxiety state. *Acta Psychiatr Scan* 1975; **51**: 69–76

21. Roth M, Gurney C, Garside RF et al. Studies in the classification of affective disorders. The relationship between anxiety states and depressive illnesses – I. *Br J Psychiatry* 1972; **121**: 147–61.

22. Breslau N, Davis GC. DSM-III Generalized anxiety disorder: an empirical investigation of more stringent criteria. *Psychiatry Res* 1985; **14**: 231–38

23. Uhlenhuth EH, Balter MB, Mellinger GD et al. Symptom checklist syndromes in the general population. *Arch Gen Psychiatry* 1983; **40**: 1167–73.

24. Faravelli C, Degl'Innocenti BG, Giardinelli L. Epidemiology of anxiety disorders in Florence. *Acta Psychiatr Scand* 1989; **79**: 308–12.

25. Wacker HR, Mullejans R. Klein KH et al. Identification of cases of anxiety disorders and affective disorders in the community according to ICD-10 and DSM-III-R using the Composite International Diagnostic Interview (CIDI). *Int J Meth Psychiatry Res* 1992; **2**: 91–100.

26. Brawman-Mintzer O, Lydiard RB. Generalized Anxiety Disorder: issues in epidemiology. *J Clin Psychiatry* 1996; **57 (suppl 7)**: 3–8.

27. Flint AJ. Epidemiology and comorbidity of anxiety disorders in the elderly. *Am J Psychiatry* 1994; **151**: 640–49.

28. Shear MK, Schulberg HC et al. Panic and generalised anxiety disorder in primary care. Presented at a meeting of the Association for Primary Care. Washington, DC, 1994.

29. Roy-Byrne P, Katon W, Broadhead WE et al. Subsyndromal ('mixed') anxiety-depression in primary care. *J Gen Intern Med* 1994; **9**: 507–12.

30. Kashani JH, Orvaschel H. Anxiety disorders in mid-adolescence: a community sample. *Am J Psychiatry* 1988; **145**: 960–64.

31. Kushner MG, Sher KJ, Beitman BD. The relation between alcohol problems and the anxiety disorders. *Am J Psychiatry* 1990; **147**: 685–95.

32. Ross HE, Glasser FB, Germanson T. The prevalence of psychiatric disorders in patients with alcohol and other drug problems. *Arch Gen Psychiatry* 1988; **45**: 1023–31.

33. Stoudemire A. Epidemiology and psychopharmacology of anxiety in medical patients. *J Clin Psychiatry* 1996; **57 (suppl 7)**: 64–72.

34. Starkstein SE, Cohen BS, Federoff FP et al. Relationship between anxiety disorders and depressive disorders in patients with cerebrovascular injury. *Arch Gen Psychiatry* 1990; **47**: 246–51.

35. Morris PL, Robinson RG, Raphael B. The prevalence and course of depressive disorders in hospitalized stroke patients. *Int J Psychiatry Med* 1990; **20**: 349–64.

36. Lydiard RB. Anxiety and the irritable bowel syndrome: Psychiatric, medical, or both? *J Clin Psychiatry* 1997; **58 (suppl 3)**: 51–58.

37. Magni G, Bernasconi G, Mauro P et al. Psychiatric diagnoses in ulcerative colitis. *Br J Psychiatry* 1991; **158**: 413–15.

38. Lustman PJ, Griffith LS, Clouse RE et al. Psychiatric illness in diabetes mellitus: relationship to symptoms and glucose control. *J Nerv Ment Dis* 1986; **174**: 736–42.

39. Fischler B, Cluydts R, de Gucht V et al. Generalised anxiety disorder in chronic fatigue syndrome. *Acta Psychiatr Scand* 1997; **95**: 405–13.

40. Brown TA, Barlow DH, Liebowitz MR. The empirical basis of generalized anxiety disorder. *Am J Psychiatry* 1994; **151**: 1272–80.

41. Bienvenu OJ, Nestadt G, Eaton WW. Characterising generalized anxiety: temporal and symptomatic thresholds. *J Nerv Ment Dis* 1998; **186**: 51–56.

42. Kendler KS, Neale MC, Kessler RC et al. Clinical characteristics of familial generalized anxiety disorder. *Anxiety* 1994/1995; **1**: 186–91.

43. Keller MB, Lavori PW, Wunder J et al. Chronic course of anxiety disorders in children and adolescents. *J Am Acad Child Adolesc Psychiatry* 1992; **31**: 595–99.

44. Yonkers KA, Warsaw MG, Massion AO et al. Phenomenology and course of generalised anxiety disorder. *Br J Psychiatry* 1996; **168**: 308–13.

45. Schweizer E. Generalized anxiety disorder: longitudinal course and pharmacologic treatment. *Psychiatr Clin North Am* 1995; **18**: 843–57.

46. Taylor S, Livesley WJ. The influence of personality on the clinical course of neurosis. *Curr Opin Psychiatry* 1995; **8:** 93–97.

47. Reich JM, Vasile RG. Effect of personality disorders on the treatment outcome of Axis I conditions: an update. *J Nerv Ment Dis* 1993; **181**: 475–84.

48. Sangal R, Coyle G. Chronic anxiety and social adjustment. *Compr Psychiatry* 1983; **24**: 75–78.

49. Hoehn-Saric R. Characteristics of chronic anxiety patients. In: Klein DF, Rablin J, eds. Anxiety: *New Research and Changing Concepts*. New York, NY: Raven Press, 1981.

50. Nisita C, Petracca A, Akiskal HS et al. Delinitation of generalized anxiety disorder: clinical comparisons with panic and major depressive disorders. *Compr Psychiatry* 1990; **31**: 409–15.

51. Massion AO, Warshaw MG, Keller MB. Quality of life and psychiatric morbidity in panic disorder and generalized anxiety disorder. *Am J Psychiatry* 1993; **150**: 600–07.

52. Du Pont RL, Rice DP, Miller LS et al. Economic costs of anxiety disorders. *Anxiety* 1996; **2**: 167–72.

53. Fifer SK, Mathias SD, Patrick DL et al. Untreated anxiety among adult primary care patients in a health maintenance organisation. *Arch Gen Psychiatry* 1994; **51**: 740–50.

54. Clancy J, Noyes R Jr. Anxiety neurosis: a disease for the medical model. *Psychosomatics* 1976; **17**: 90–93.

55. Katon W, von Korff M, Lin E et al. Distressed high utilisers of medical care: DSM-III-R diagnoses and treatment needs. *Gen Hosp Psychiatry* 1990; **12**: 355–62.

56. Torgersen S. Genetic factors in anxiety disorders. *Arch Gen Psychiatry* 1983; **40**: 1085–89.

57. Andrews G, Stewart G, Allen R, Henderson AS. The genetics of six neurotic disorders: a twin study. *J Affect Disord* 1990; **19**: 23–29.

58. Skre I, Onstad S, Torgensen S et al. A twin study of DSM-III-R anxiety disorders. *Acta Psychiat Scand* 1993; **88**: 85–92.

59. Noyes R Jr, Clarkson C, Crowe RR et al. A family study of generalized anxiety disorder. *Am J Psychiatry* 1987; **144**: 1019–24.

60. Scherrer JF, True WR, Xian H et al. Evidence for genetic influences common and specific to symptoms of generalised anxiety and panic. *J Affect Disord* 2000; **57**: 25–35.

61. Kendler KS, Walters EE, Neale MC et al. The structure of the genetic and environmental risk factors for six major psychiatric disorders in women: phobia, generalized anxiety disorder, panic disorder, bulimia, major depression, and alcoholism. *Arch Gen Psychiatry* 1995; **52**: 374–83.

62. Lesch K-P, Bengal D, Heils A et al. Association of anxiety-related traits with a polymorphism in the serotonin transporter gene regulatory region. *Science* 1996; **274**: 1527–31.

63. Brawman-Mintzer O, Lydiard RB. Biological basis of generalized anxiety disorder. *J Clin Psychiatry* 1997; **58 (suppl 3)**: 16–25.

64. Wu JC, Buchsbaum MS, Hershey TG et al. PET in generalized anxiety disorder. *Biol Psychiatry* 1991; **29**: 1181–99.

65. Buchsbaum MS, Wu J, Haier R et al. Positron emission tomography assessment of the effect of benzodiazepines on regional glucose metabolic rate in patients with anxiety disorder. *Life Sci* 1987; **40**: 2393–2400.

66. Nutt DJ. Neurobiological mechanisms in generalized anxiety disorder. *J Clin Psychiatry* 2001; in press.

67. Cowey DS, Roy-Byrne PP, Hommer DW et al. Benzodiazepine sensitivity in anxiety disorders. *Biol Psychiatry* 1991; **29**: 57A.

68. Weizman R, Tanne Z, Granek M et al. Peripheral benzodiazepine binding sites on platelet membranes are increased during diazepam treatment of anxious patients. *Eur J Pharmacol* 1987; **138**: 289–92.

69. Ferrarese C. Appollonio I, Frigo M et al. Decreased density of benzodiazepine receptors in lymphocytes of anxious patients: reversal after chronic diazepam treatment. *Acta Psychiatr Scand* 1990; **82**: 169–73.

70. Tiihonen J, Kuikka J, Rasansen P et al. Cerebral benzodiazepine receptor binding and distribution in generalized anxiety disorder: a fractal analysis. *Mol Psychiatry* 1997; **2**: 463–71.

71. Malizia AL, Cunningham VJ, Bell CJ et al. Decreased brain GABA (A)-benzodiazepine receptor binding in panic disorder: preliminary results from a quantitative PET study. *Arch Gen Psychiatry* 1998; **55**: 715–20.

72. Tokunga M, Ida I, Higuchi T, Mikuni M. Alterations of benzodiazepine receptor binding potential in anxiety and somatoform disorders measured by ^{123}I-lomazenil SPECT. *Rad Medicine* 1997; **15**: 163–9.

73. Deakin JFW, Graeff FG. 5-HT and mechanisms of defence. *J Psychopharmacol* 1991; 305–15.

74. Lucki I. Serotonin receptor specificity in anxiety disorders. *J Clin Psychiatry* 1996; **57 (suppl 6)**: 5–10.

75. Brewerton TD, Lydiard RB, Johnson MR et al. CFS serotonin: diagnostic and seasonal differences. In: *New research and abstracts of the 148th meeting of the American Psychiatric Association*; Miami, Fla, 1995, Abstract NR385:151.

76. Germine M. Goddard AW, Woods SW et al. Anger and anxiety responses to m-chlorophenylpiperazine in generalized anxiety disorder. *Biol Psychiatry* 1992; **32**: 457–61.

77. Charney DS, Nagy LM, Bremner JD et al. Neurobiological mechanisms of human anxiety. In Fogel BS, Schiffer RB, Rao SM, eds. *Neuropsychiatry*. Baltimore: Williams & Wilkins, 1996: 257–86.

78. Matthew RJ, Ho BT, Francis DJ et al. Catecholamines and anxiety. *Acta Psychiatr Scand* 1992; **65**: 142–47.

79. Kelly CB, Cooper SJ. Differences in variability in plasma noradrenaline between depressive and anxiety disorders. *J Psychopharmacol* 1998; **12**: 161–67.

80. Khan A, Lee E, Dager S et al. Platelet MAO-B activity in anxiety and depression. *Biol Psychiatry* 1986; **21**: 847–49.

81. Abelson JL, Glitz D, Cameron OG et al. Blunted growth hormone response to clonidine in patients with generalized anxiety disorder. *Arch Gen Psychiatry* 1991; **48**: 157–62.

82. Hoehn-Saric R, McLeod DR, Zimmerli WD, Somatic manifestations in women with generalized anxiety disorder. *Arch Gen Psychiatry* 1989; **46**: 1113–19.

83. Thayer JF, Friedman BH, Borcovec TD. Autonomic characteristics of generalized anxiety disorder and worry. *Biol Psychiatry* 1996; **39**: 255–66.

84. Marten PA, Brown TA, Barlow DH et al. Evaluation of the ratings comprising the asscoiated symptom criterion of DSM-III-R generalized anxiety disorder. *J Nerv Ment Diseases* 1994; **181**: 676–82.

85. Hoehn-Saric R, Hazlett RL. Pourmotabbed T, McLeod DR. Does muscle tension reflect arousal? Relationship between electromyographic and electroencephalographic recordings. *Psych Research* 1997; **71**: 49–55.

86. Saletu-Zyhlarz G, Saletu B, Anderer P et al. Nonorganic insomnia in generalized anxiety disorder. 1. Controlled studies of sleep, awakening and daytime vigilance utilising polysomnography and EEG mapping. *Neuropsychobiology* 1997; **36**: 117–29.

87. Reynolds CF III, Shaw DH, Newton TF et al. EEG sleep in outpatients with generalized anxiety: a preliminary comparison with depressed outpatients. *Psych Research* 1983; **8**: 81–9.

88. Gray JA. The neuropsychological basis of anxiety. In: Last CG, Hersen M, eds. *Handbook of Anxiety Disorders*. New York: Pergamon Press, 1988: 10–37.

89. Bowlby J. Attachment and loss, Vol II: *Separation, anxiety and anger*. London: Hogarth Press, 1973.

90. Bowlby J. The making and breaking of affectional bonds. *Br J Psychiatry* 1977; **130**: 201–10.

91. Parker G. *Parental overprotection, a risk for psychosocial development*. New York: Grune and Stratton, 1983.

92. Parker G, Tupling H, Brown LB et al. The Parental Bonding Instrument. *Br J Med Psychol* 1979; **52**: 1–10.

93. Parker G. Reported parental characteristics in relation to trait depression and anxiety levels in a non clinical group. *Aust N Z J Psychiatry* 1979; **13**: 260–64.

94. Parker G. Validating an experimental measure of parental style: the use of a twin sample. *Acta Psychiatr Scand* 1986; **73**: 22–27.

95. Silove D, Parker G, Hadzi-Pavlovic D et al. Parental representations of patients with panic disorder and generalised anxiety disorder. *Br J Psychiatry* 1991; **159**: 835–41.

96. Torgersen S. Childhood and family characteristics in panic and generalized anxiety disorders. *Am J Psychiatry* 1986; **143**: 630–32.

97. Blazer D, Hughes D, George LK. Stressful life events and the onset of a generalized anxiety syndrome. *Am J Psychiatry* 1987; **144**: 1178–83.

98. Steketee G, Foa EB. Rape victims: post traumatic stress responses and their treatment: a review of the literature. *J Anx Disorders* 1987; **1**: 69–86.

99. Roemer L, Molina S, Litz BT et al. Preliminary investigation of the role of previous exposure to potentially traumatising events in generalized anxiety disorder. *Depr Anxiety* 1996/1997; **4**: 134–38.

100. Brown GW, Harris TO, Eales MJ. Social factors and comorbidity of depressive and anxiety disorders. *Br J Psychiatry* 1996; **168 (suppl 30)**: 50–57.

101. Finlay-Jones R. Anxiety. In: Brown GW, Harris TO, eds. *Life events and illness. Vol 1*. New York: Guildford Press, 1989: 95–112.

102. Beck AT, Emery G. *Anxiety disorders and phobia: a cognitive perspective*. New York: Basic Books, 1985.

103. Butler G, Fennell M, Robson P et al. Comparison of behaviour therapy and cognitive behaviour therapy in the treatment of generalized anxiety disorder. *J Consult Clin Psychol* 1991; **59**: 167–75.

104. Borkovec TD, Shadick R, Hopkins M. The nature of normal and pathological worry in chronic anxiety: generalized

anxiety disorder and mixed anxiety depression. Rapee RM, Barlow DH, eds. New York: Guildford Press, 1991: 29–51.

105. Matthews A, Macleod C. Selective processing of threat cues in anxiety states. *Behav Res Ther* 1985; **23**: 536–69.

106. Bradley BP, Mogg K, White J et al. Attentional bias for emotional faces in generalized anxiety disorder. *Br J Clin Psychology* 1999; **38**: 267–78.

107. Hoehn-Saric R, Macleod DR. The peripheral sympathetic nervous system: its role in normal and pathological anxiety. *Psychiatr Clin North Am* 1988; **11**: 375–86.

108. Roemer L, Borkovec TD. Worry: unwanted cognitive experience that controls unwanted somatic experince. In Wegner DM, Pennebaker J, eds. *Handbook of mental control.* Englewood Cliffs, N.J: Prentice Hall, 1993.

109. Borkovec TD. The nature, functions and origins of worry. In: Davey GCL, Tallis F, eds. *Worrying: perspectives in theory, assessment and treatment.* England: John Wiley & Sons, 1994.

110. Harvey AG, Rapee RM. Cognitive-behaviour therapy for generalized anxiety disorder. *Psychiatr Clin North Am* 1995; **18**: 859–70.

111. Durham RC, Allan T. Psychological treatment of generalised anxiety disorder. A review of the clinical significance of results in outcome studies since 1980. *Br J Psychiatry* 1993; **163**: 19–26.

112. Hunt C. The diagnosis and nature of generalized anxiety disorder. *Cur Op Psychiatry* 2000; **13**: 157–61.

113. Molina S, Borkovec TD, Peasley C, Person D. Content analysis of worrisome streams of consciousness in anxious and dysphoric participants. *Cogn Ther Res* 1998; **22**: 109-23.

114. Borkovec TD, Ray WJ, Stoeber J. Worry: a cognitive phenomenon intimately linked to affective, physiological, and interpersonal behavioral processes. *Cogn Ther Res* 1998; **22**: 561–76.

115. Wells A, Carter K. Preliminary tests of a cognitive model of generalized anxiety disorder. *Behav Res Ther* 1999; **37**: 585–94.

116. Davey GCL, Levy S. Catastrophic worrying: personal inadequacy and a perseverative iterative style as features of the catastrophising process. *J Abnorm Psychol* 1998; **107**: 576–86.

117. Dugas MJ, Gagnon F, Ladoucer R, Freeston MH. Generalized anxiety disorder: a preliminary test of a conceptual model. *Behav Res Ther* 1998; **36**: 215–26.

118. Kessler RC, Nelson CB, McGonagle KA et al. Comorbidity of DSM-III-R major depressive disorder in the general population: results from the US National Comorbidity Survey. *Br J Psychiatry* 1996; **168 (suppl 30)**: 17–30.

119. Goldberg D. A dimensional model for common mental disorders. *Br J Psychiatry* 1996; **168 (suppl 30)**: 44–49.

120. Gorman JM. Cormorbid depression and anxiety spectrum disorders. *Depr Anxiety* 1996/1997; **4**: 160–68.

121. Piccinelli M. Comorbidity of depression and generalized anxiety: is there any distinct boundary? *Curr Opin Psychiatry* 1998; **11**: 57–60.

122. Stahl SM. Mixed depression and anxiety: serotonin 1A receptors as a common pharmacologic link. *J Clin Psychiatry* 1997; **58 (suppl 8)**: 20–26.

123. Kendler KS. Major depression and generalised anxiety disorder. Some genes, (partly) different environments - revisited. *Br J Psychiatry* 1996; **168 (suppl 30)**: 68–75.

124. Marks I. Agoraphobia, panic disorder and related conditions in the DSM-III-R and ICD-10. *J Psychopharmacol* 1987; **1**: 6–12.

125. Tyrer P. Classification of anxiety disorders. *J Affect Disorders* 1986; **11**: 99–104.

126. Garvey MJ, Cook B, Noyes R Jr. The occurrence of a prodrome of generalised anxiety in panic disorder. *Compr Psychiatry* 1988; **29**: 445–449.

127. Fava GA. Grandi S, Canestrari R. Prodromal symptoms in panic disorder with agoraphobia. *Am J Psychiatry* 1988; **12:** 1564–1567.

128. Breier A, Charney DS, Heninger GR. Agoraphobia with panic attacks. *Arch Gen Psychiatry* 1986, **43**: 1029–1036.

129. Crowe RR, Noyes R Jr, Pauls DL, Slymen D. A family study of panic disorder. *Arch Gen Psychiatry* 1983; **40**: 1065–1069.

130. Noyes R Jr, Crowe RR, Harris EL et al. Relationship between panic disorder and agoraphobia: a family study. *Arch Gen Psychiatry* 1986; **43**: 227–232.

131. Noyes R Jr, Woodman C, Garvey MJ et al. Generalized anxiety disorder vs panic disorder. Distinguishing characteristics and patterns of comorbidity. *J Nerv Ment Diseases* 1992; **180**: 369–379.

132. Breitholtz E, Johansson B, Ost LG. Cognitions in generalized anxiety disorder and panic disorder patients. A prospective approach. *Behav Res Ther* 1999; **37**: 533–44.

133. Verburg K, Griex E, Meijer J et al. Discrimination between panic disorder and generalised anxiety disorder by 35% carbon dioxide challenge. *Am J Psychiatry* 1995; **152**: 1081–1083.

134. Black DW, Goldstein RB, Noyes R Jr, Blum N. Psychiatric disorders in relatives of probands with obsessive-compulsive disorder and co-morbid major depression or generalized anxiety. *Psych Genetics* 1995; **5**: 37–41.

135. Andrews G, Stewart G, Morris-Yates A et al. Evidence for a general neurotic syndrome. *Br J Psychiatry* 1990; **157**: 6–12.

136. Roemer L, Molina S, Borcovec TD. An investigation of worry contents among generally anxious individuals. *J Nerv Ment Disorders* 1997; **185**: 314–319.

137. Steketee GS, Grayson JB, Foa EB. A comparison of characteristics of obsessive-compulsive disorder and other anxiety disorders. *J Anx Disorders* 1987; **1**: 325–335.

138. Tallis F, DeSilva P. Worry and obsessional symptoms: a correlational analysis. *Behav Res Therapy* 1992; **30**: 103–105.

139. Nutt DJ, Bell CJ, Potokar JP. Drug-treatment of chronic anxiety. *Balliere's Clin Psychiatry* 1995; **1**: 565–94.

140. Rickels K, Schweizer E. Benzodiazepines for the treatment of panic attacks: A new look. *Psychopharmacol Bull* 1986; **22**: 93–99.

141. Rickels K, Schweizer E, Case GC and Greenblatt DJ. Long-term therapeutic use of benzodiazepines: I. Effects of abrupt discontinuation. *Arch Gen Psychiatry* 1990; **47**: 899–907.

142. Schweizer E, Rickels K, Case GC et al. Lon-term therapeutic use of benzodiazepines: II. Effects of gradual taper. *Arch Gen Psychiatry* 1990; **47**: 908–15.

143. Nutt DJ. The psychopharmacology of anxiety. *Br J Hosp Med* 1996; **55**: 187–91.

144. Delle Chiaie R, Pancheri P, Casacchia M et al. Assessment of the efficacy of buspirone in patients affected by generalized anxiety disorder, shifting to buspirone from prior treatment with lorazepam: a placebo-controlled, double-blind study. *J Clin Psychopharmacol* 1995; **15**: 12–19.

145. Kahn RJ, McNair DM, Lipman RS et al. Imipramine and chlordiazepoxide in depressive and anxiety disorders: Efficacy in anxious outpatients. *Arch Gen Psychiatry* 1986; **43**: 79–85.

146. Rickels K. Downing R, Schweizer E, Hassman H. Antidepressants for the treatment of generalized anxiety disorder. *Arch Gen Psychiatry* 1993; **50**: 884–95.

147. Rudolph RL, Entsuah R, Chitra R. A meta-analysis of the effects of venlafaxine on anxiety associated with depression. *J Clin Psychopharmacol* 1998; **18**: 136–44.

148. Rickels K, Pollack MH, Sheehan DV, Haskins JT. Efficacy of extended-release venlafaxine in nondepressed outpatients with generalized anxiety disorder. *Am J Psychiatry* 2000; **157**: 968–74.

149. Davidson JRT, DuPont RL, Hedges D, Haskins JT. Efficacy, safety, and tolerability of venlafaxine extended release and buspirone in outpatients with generalised anxiety disorder. *J Clin Psychiatry* 1999; **60**: 528–35.

150. Gelenberg AJ, Lydiard RB, Rudolph RL et al. Efficacy of venlafaxine extended-release capsules in nondepressed outpatients with generalized anxiety disorder. A 6-month randomised controlled trial. *JAMA* 2000; **283**: 3082–88.

151. Pollack MH, Zanielli R, Goddard A et al. Paroxetine in the treatment of Generalized Anxiety Disorder: results of a placebo-controlled, flexible-dosage trial. *J Clin Psychiatry* 2001; **62**: in press.

152. Stocchi F, Nordera G, Jokinen R et al. Efficacy and tolerability of paroxetine for the long-term treatment of generalized anxiety disorder (GAD). Poster presented at the 154th annual meeting of the American Psychiatric Association, New Orleans, USA, 6–10 May, 2001.

153. Weiss BL. Controlled comparison of trifluoperazine and chlordiazepoxide in the treatment of anxiety. *Curr Ther Res* 1997; **22**: 635–43.

154. Wurthmann C, Klieser E, Lehman E. Side effects of low dose neuroleptics and their impact on clinical outcome in generalized anxiety disorder. *Prog Neuropsychopharm Biol Psychiatry* 1997; **21**: 601–09.

155. El-Khayat R. Baldwin D. Antipsychotic drugs for non-psychotic patients: assessment of the benefit/risk ratio in generalised anxiety disorder. *J Psychopharmacol* 1998; **12**: 323–29.

156. Ferreri M, Hantouche E-G. Recent clinical trials of hydroxyzine in generalised anxiety disorder. *Acta Psychiatr Scand* 1998; **98 (suppl 393)**: 102–08.

157. Bell CJ, Nutt DJ. Serotonin and panic. *Br J Psychiatry* 1998; **172**: 465–71.

158. Dar R. Treatment of obsessive-compulsive disorder. *Curr Opinion Psychiatr* 1996; **9**: 125–8.

159. Kunovac JL, Stahl SM. Future directions in anxiolytic pharmacotherapy. *Psychiatr Clin North Am* 1995; **18**: 895–909.

160. Lydiard RB, Ballenger JC, Rickels K. A double-blind evaluation of the safety and efficacy of abercanil, alprazolam and placebo in outpatients with generalized anxiety disorder. *J Clin Psychiatry* 1997; **58 (suppl 11)**: 11–18.

161. Rickels K, Schweizer E, De Martinis N et al. Gepirone and diazepam in generalized anxiety disorders: a placebo-controlled trial. *J Clin Psychopharmacol* 1997; **17**: 272–77.

162. Katz RJ, Landau PS Lott M et al. Serotonergic (5-HT2) mediation of anxiety–therapeutic effects of serazepine in generalized anxiety disorder. *Biol Psychiatry* 1993; **34**: 41–44.

163. Freeman AM, Westphal JR, Norris GT et al. Efficacy of ondansetron in the treatment of generalized anxiety disorder. *Depr Anxiety* 1997; **5**: 140–41.

164. Bammert Adams J, Pyke RE, Costa J et al. A double-blind, placebo-controlled study of a CCK-B receptor antagonist, CI-988, in patients with generalized anxiety disorder. *J Clin Psychopharmacol* 1995; **15**: 428–34.

165. Schweitzer E, Rickels K. The long-term management of generalized anxiety disorder: issues and dilemmas. *J Clin Psychiatry* 1996; **57 (suppl 7)**: 9–14.

166. Rickels K, Schweizer E. The clinical presentation of generalized anxiety in primary-care settings: practical concepts of classification and management. *J Clin Psychiatry* 1997; **58 (suppl 11)**: 4–10.

167. Hollander E, Cohen LJ. The assessment and treatment of refractory anxiety. *J Clin Psychiatry* 1994; **55 (suppl 2)**: 27–31.

168. Jannoun L, Oppenheimer C, Gelder M. A self-help treatment program for anxiety. *Behav Res Ther* 1982; **13**: 103–11.

169. Butler G, Cullington A, Hibbert G. Anxiety management for persistent generalised anxiety state patients. *Br J Psychiatry* 1987; **151**: 535–42.

170. Barlow DH. Anxiety and its disorders. The nature and treatment of anxiety and panic. New York: Guildford Press, 1988.

171. Durham RC, Murphy T, Allan T et al. Cognitive therapy, analytic psychotherapy and anxiety management training for generalised anxiety disorder. *Br J Psychiatry* 1994; **165**: 315–23.

172. Borkovec TD, Costello E. Efficacy of applied relaxation and cognitive behavioural therapy in the treatment of generalized anxiety disorder. *J Consult Clin Psychol* 1993; **61**: 611–19.

173. Durham RC, Turvey AA. Cognitive therapy vs. behaviour therapy in the treatment of chronic generalised anxiety. *Behav Res Ther* 1987; **25**: 229–34.

174. Lindsay W, Gamsu C, McLaughlin E et al. A controlled trial of treatments for generalised anxiety. *Br J Clin Psychol* 1987; **2**: 3–15.

175. Borkovec TD, Whisman MA. Psychosocial treatment for generalized anxiety disorder. In: Mavissakalian MR, Prien RF, eds. *Long-term treatments of anxiety disorders.* Washington DC: American Psychiatric Press, 1996: 171–99.

176. Power KG. A controlled comparison of cognitive-behavioral therapy, diazepam, and placebo, alone and in combination, for the treatment of generalised anxiety disorder. *J Anx Disord* 1990; **4**: 535–42.

177. Raskin M, Bali L, Peeke H. Muscle biofeedback and transcendental meditation: a controlled evaluation of efficacy in the treatment of chronic anxiety. *Arch Gen Psychiatry* 1980; **37**: 93–97.

178. Kingdon D, Tyrer P, Seivewright N et al. The Nottingham study of neurotic disorder: influence of cognitive therapists on outcome. *Br J Psychiatry* 1996; **169**: 93–7.

179. Beck AT, Freeman A. *Cognitive therapy of personality disorders.* New York: Guildford Press, 1990.

Index

GAD = generalized anxiety disorder
OCD = obsessive-compulsive disorder
SSRIs = serotonin reuptake inhibitors